JUDITH HANN'S TOTAL HEALTH PLAN is based
on a simple but intelligent routine which is so easy and
painless to follow that it soon becomes a way of life.
And it is a way of life which is far healthier, with its
minimal changes in eating, vitamin intake, exercise and
alcohol consumption, than extreme habits like dieting,
weight lifting and marathon running.

EXTREME DIETS can slow down your body
metabolism so that when you begin to eat normally
again you quickly put on more weight than ever before.
Spurning alcohol might be good for the soul, but
research has shown that your arteries are healthier if you
enjoy a couple of glasses of wine, or the equivalent,
each day. Extreme vitamin regimes can lead to
dangerous, long-term overdosing. Over-vigorous
exercise can lead to bone damage, infertility, and fatal
heart attacks.

MANY PEOPLE want and need to have a TOTAL
HEALTH PLAN worked out for them. A plan which is
scientifically thorough, while still being realistic and
practical.

JUDITH HANN'S TOTAL HEALTH PLAN is the
easy, effortless way to good health, weight loss, general
fitness and looking and feeling great.

Judith Hann's Total Health Plan

Judith Hann

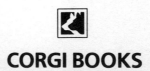

CORGI BOOKS

JUDITH HANN'S TOTAL HEALTH PLAN

A CORGI BOOK 0 552 12379 X

First publication in Great Britain

PRINTING HISTORY
Corgi edition published 1984

This book is set in 10/11 Century Textbook

Corgi Books are published by
Transworld Publishers Ltd.,
Century House, 61–63 Uxbridge Road,
Ealing, London W5 5SA

Made and printed in Great Britain by
Cox & Wyman Ltd., Reading, Berks.

Contents

Introduction   7
1 Judith Hann's Total Health Plan   8
2 The Total Food Plan   16
   My Simple Plan Simplified   18
   A Day in the Total Health Plan   21
   Avoiding Obesity and Disease with
      the Total Health Plan   22
   The Total Food Plan Explained   25
   Healthy Cooking Methods   33
   Royal College of Physician's 'Obesity'
      Report   36
   Postscript   38
3 The Total Exercise Plan   40
   The Total Exercise Plan Explained   43
4 The Drinking Plan   59
5 The Vitamin Plan   62
6 The Anti-Stress Plan   71
7 Cooking for Health — A Few Recipes for
      the Total Health Plan   76
8 Shopping for Total Health   93
9 Aerobic Exercises at Home   98
10 One Week in My Total Health Plan   105

Introduction

A year ago I was almost forty and weighed almost 11 stone. It was not a happy combination for someone who had spent the first half of her life as a lean, lithe and lively individual.

I was not really tempted to give in to middle-age, and accept its well-documented 'spread'. It was partly self-respect, and partly my suspicion that we have no excuse for becoming less healthy as we age.

When I began to research the whole subject of health and lifestyle, I was swamped by vast numbers of 'miracle' cures, which promised loss of weight, perfect bodies and extra vitality. They were, inevitably, not only useless but dangerous because they attracted desperate people who wanted to solve difficult personal problems, and who fanatically followed the latest fashionable regime, only to become obsessed by something which would ultimately fail.

The real answer to being healthy, whatever your age, is very different. After sifting through the scientific studies on this subject, I have compiled a Total Health Plan which is far from obsessive. It is simple to understand, and easy to put into practice. And it works. There is no point in dieting. There are disadvantages in extreme exercise. This is a health plan which you can read in one evening, and then use to change your whole life without really trying.

It has certainly changed mine. I have lost over 16 pounds, and gained a lot of vitality. Do the same by following my simple rules for eating, exercising, drinking, taking vitamins and avoiding stress. Modify your life — and enjoy it more. This Total Health Plan really is the way to live longer, without killing yourself.

1 Judith Hann's Total Health Plan

I plan to live longer without killing myself. And after reading my Total Health Plan I am sure that you will do the same, realising that you can become healthier, slimmer and fitter with very little effort. You will find the plan so easy and painless to follow that it will soon become a way of life.

It is a way of life which is FAR HEALTHIER, with its MINIMAL changes in eating, exercise, vitamin intake and alcohol consumption, than EXTREME habits like severe dieting and long distance running. Health fanatics may get a psychological kick out of obsessively following their chosen, rigid regime, but it is all too often bad for them physically.

Dieting, for example, slows down your body metabolism, so that when you begin to eat normally again you soon put on more weight than ever before. Spurning alcohol might be good for the soul, but research has shown that your arteries could be healthier if you enjoy a couple of glasses of wine, or the equivalent, each day. Extreme vitamin regimes can lead to dangerous overdosing, while just a few of the scientifically-sound vitamins might work wonders. Over-vigorous exercise can lead to bone damage, infertility and fatal heart attacks.

I could go on. But to sum up, health is one area of your life where MAKING LESS EFFORT CAN BE GOOD FOR YOU.

If you do a LITTLE of the right things you achieve a LOT. While if you do a LOT within one fanatical regime, you achieve LITTLE.

I decided to formulate the Total Health Plan after talking to scientists working in this field, reading research papers on health, and actually taking part in some of the health projects over a period of three years. I was finally ready to put my conclusions into practice a year ago, appropriately, at about the time I had my fortieth birthday. Now, after those twelve months of slightly modifying my eating and drinking, while following a simple exercise plan, I am one stone lighter without dieting at all. And, although I have not pushed myself in any way, I am fitter and livelier than I have been for years.

My friends have noticed the difference, so they have been asking me for the secret. Their interest has convinced me that there are a vast number of people in Britain who now want and need to have a simple health plan worked out for them, which is scientifically thorough, while still being realistic and practical.

The main difficulty for anyone reading magazine and newspaper articles about the latest scientific conclusions on certain foods, vitamins or exercise regimes, is that it is often impossible for the layman to understand and apply those conclusions to everyday life. I am asked, for example, what recent research on dangers from dietary fats means in our kitchens. How much animal fat can we have a day without being at risk? Which are the safest cooking oils? Should we use low-fat or polyunsaturated fat spreads? And I find that people are just as confused by conflicting scientific research on jogging and other forms of exercise. Will running lengthen or shorten my life, they ask?

It is not surprising that people are muddled, because many of the scientists themselves have been muddled for years. And it is also not surprising that so many people in Britain are sceptical about health ideas. We have been bombarded with dozens of anti-ageing and pro-fitness notions that have ultimately turned out to be absolute nonsense. No wonder the term 'Health

Food Nut' was coined. This whole area is full of fads, fanatics and fakes.

At the start of my research, I was as confused and sceptical as anybody else, despite my interest in the science of health, developed over twenty years as a science writer and television presenter. I had no blinding ambition to formulate the perfect health plan, partly because I am not a worthy do-gooder by nature and partly because I have a tendency to eat and drink too much. Like many other people in Britain, I am a little bit of a slob. I have never had the 'free-range cornflakes' mentality and I have always avoided any form of exercise I did not enjoy.

But after three years of research, I am now convinced that it is possible to firm up what has always been a flabby science. We have been getting it wrong for years, either by doing *nothing* about our health or by doing *too much*. What we should be doing is *a little*. By making MINIMAL changes in the TOTAL health area, we can quite painlessly live a healthier, fitter and longer life. Moderation in everything is the simple message.

We should have begun to make these changes a long time ago. We have a poor health record in Britain compared to most other countries. Admittedly, there have always been health enthusiasts with their own preservation techniques, from merely spreading low fat margarines, to jogging several miles a day. But they are in the minority. Most of us do very little to hang on to our health, looks and vitality.

And this shows medically. Britain has one of the highest rates for coronary heart disease in the world. Indeed, the rate in Scotland and Northern Ireland is now *the highest* in the world. Although America has reduced heart disease by 20% in the last decade, partly by lifestyle changes, like more exercise and healthier eating, we have not yet seen these improvements in Britain.

In fact, doctors in this country think the situation is

getting worse. Last year a Royal College of Physicians report on *Obesity* claimed that the number of people eating too much and exercising too little is increasing rapidly. Over one third of us are now overweight and as we increase our girth we increase our chances of getting heart disease, diabetes and some types of cancer.

Two out of five of us are likely to die from heart disease, one in five could die from cancer, and one in seven from high blood pressure. But we can do something to improve these statistics. Many Americans, Canadians, Australians, Belgians, and other Europeans have altered their lifestyles with excellent results, and so have the more highly motivated people in this country. But that still leaves the majority of us who have a tendency to be sceptical slobs.

Fortunately I have good news for them. It is much easier to be healthy than most of the experts have ever admitted. The painfully rigid dieting regimes are a waste of time for most of us. 95% of crash diets fail because the excess weight soon piles back on. Extreme exercise can be very dangerous. Excessive health regimes have been pushed by author after author. Many of the writers have been American and a good few of them have been bestsellers. But the evidence shows that people usually buy these health books because the very act of buying them makes them feel better. They think they are doing something constructive — but when they actually read the fanatical health advice, they are usually sensible enough to leave the books' ideas on their shelves. The Americans have not become healthier over the past few years by following the advice found in fashionable, faddy diet books or silly exercise manuals. It is doctors and scientists who have taken the lead, with great help from the American Heart Association. Perhaps because Americans have to pay for their health care, they have listened to what the experts have to say and they have modified their lifestyle.

We should now do the same. First we need to ignore the fashionable, excessive regimes which regularly find their way to Britain from America, like the Pineapple Diet, the Green Diet and so on. These books should be left in mid-Atlantic. Britain needs a national campaign in which doctors and scientists address the nation directly, as has been done in America. I believe this will happen soon.

The 1983 report by the National Advisory Committee on Nutrition Education, a Government appointed committee of food experts who issued, *Proposals for Nutritional Guidelines for Health Education in Britain*, helped to stimulate interest. (Report issued by the Health Education Council) After reading it many people began to agree that perhaps the typical British diet should carry a Government Health warning. The report claimed that we eat too much fat, too much sugar and salt, and too little fibre. When it was published I had been following my Total Health Plan for over a year, and it recommended much the same long-term goals: reducing fat to 30% of our total energy intake, increasing fibre by a third, and reducing salt to half or even a quarter of our present intake. In the short-term, the report suggested smaller changes to allow for difficult adjustments.

The next aim of many nutrition experts is to persuade the Government to develop a policy on nutrition, so that the public would be given sensible advice on the foods to eat. They believe, as I do, that it is less important to wait for *absolute* proof on safe salt levels or the dangers of all types or fat, for example, than to give the *best* advice that we have at the *moment*, which could begin to save lives now.

Perhaps in the future the Government will insist that the Milk Marketing Board provides low-fat milk, that cheese is labelled for fat content, that wholemeal bread becomes cheaper and that there is less sugar and salt in processed foods. But until then we have to make our own decisions. This can be done easily by following the advice in this book which uses internationally agreed goals, including reducing fat intake, trying to cut sugar and salt by half, eating more fibre, fresh fruit and vegetables, while exercising aerobically for one hour a week.

After incorporating these goals into my own life-style for one year, I can guarantee that my Total Health Plan is easy to follow, particularly if the minor changes are introduced gradually. Even slobs will find it relatively easy to change their ways. And they will soon feel so much better that they will not be tempted to revert to their old, bad habits.

Smoking is not mentioned in my plan because I assume that everyone now accepts the evidence that cigarettes are dangerous. Food is a more complicated story, but luckily the evidence has firmed up recently and there are now sensible guidelines to follow. I have found it a challenge to formulate a friendly, sociable food plan, which is scientifically sound. And I have been gratified to find that the new, healthier way of eating is much cheaper. With less expensive meat, and more seasonal, bargain vegetables and fruits, you can save a lot of money. This is particularly important for teenagers and people in their early twenties, who realise the need to eat in a different way to their parents. They can buy healthier foods without resorting to expensive health food stores. Market stalls have some of the cheapest and freshest of vegetables. And, as my shopping section at the back of the book shows, supermarkets are now selling most of the healthiest foods, like wholemeal pasta, low-sugar jams and cooking oils high in polyunsaturates, at the most competitive prices.

Try to keep the ten food commandments, without feeling neurotic if you break one of them occasionally. And do remember that scientists have recently warned that it is not sensible to be as skinny as many fashion models. The Ideal Weight Charts, drawn up for Life Insurance use, but also relied on by doctors and the general public, have been proved wrong. They are 5 to 10 lbs too low for each 'ideal weight', according to new research linking weight to longevity. So a little extra padding could help us to live longer — it usually makes us look more attractive too.

But this does not mean that we should overeat. We have got to be careful and thoughtful enough to keep to the rules. For example, the man who said to me: 'My wife has a good way with left-overs. . . . She chucks them into the rubbish bin,' is right. Let the left-over potatoes go to waste, because if you fry them up in fat for breakfast, they will go to waist instead.

Do resist the rubbish foods too, the junk foods which are full of empty calories. Keep sugary drinks, sweet biscuits and fatty chips out of your home. It is the only way to resist them. If they are in the kitchen, perhaps for your children, you will be tempted to eat them. And when you *eat* empty calories you *wear* them, and all their attendant health problems.

Fill your home instead with the healthy foods you really enjoy. If, perhaps, you have a passion for peaches, surround yourself with the freshest, most delicious peaches of the highest quality. They will help you to lose your taste for unhealthy chips and hamburgers. Remind yourself that they are cheaper than most junk foods.

You will find your body slowly changes to match the food you give it. But food and nutrients are only half the story. The use you make of your body is the other half and, if your normal way of life is not active, you will need to organise some exercise yourself. My ten commandments show you how to spend one hour a week on exercises ideal for your body and your interests. The Total Health Plan is simple to understand and easy to follow. Science has at last come to some firm conclusions about health and these have all been incorporated into my message. Even the most dedicated slobs need to accept that WE CAN

ALL LIVE LONGER WITHOUT KILLING
OURSELVES.

2 The Total Food Plan

THE TEN FOOD COMMANDMENTS

1. Avoid fashionable crash diets. They are unhealthy and fattening.

2. Eat double the quantity of unrefined carbo-hydrates.

3. Decrease the fat in your diet by 25%.

4. Eat less protein, especially meat.

5. Reduce salt.

6. Go easy on the sugar.

7. Try healthier cooking methods.

8. Eat a third more fresh fruit and vegetables.

9. Increase fibre. Beans and pulses are good for you.

10. Eat a wide variety of food, washed down with two glasses of wine, or the equivalent, a day. Alcohol is good for your arteries and your stress levels.

The greatest challenge in doing this book was to work out a sensible, healthy way of eating that was neither boring nor obsessive. We all need, more than ever before, an enjoyable diet that is easy to live with.

Fortunately for us all, my research has concluded that the scientifically-ideal diet allows adequate alcohol for social lubrication, copes with occasional indulgences, and encourages dinner parties with food that no keen cook would feel ashamed of. I can promise you that my eating plan does not force down so many lentils and beans that the bottom will fall out of your world because you can't stop the world falling out of your bottom. It is realistic and so simple to live with that you will soon have changed your style of eating without having to give it a great deal of thought.

Many people are now ready to give up the crazy notion of dieting and to make *smaller* changes over a *wider* food area instead. I was encouraged to hear two hardened (and overweight) dieters in my office discussing their mutual problem the other day. For the first time ever, instead of arguing the merits of the grapefruit or the high-protein diet, for example, they claimed they would never diet again. They had learnt from experience that they always put back on the pounds lost during two or three tense, hungry and depressing weeks of self-denial. 'The only way to lose weight is slowly,' said one of them. They now eat more healthily, they exercise more and they don't slop around the office. I am sure you have noticed that overweight people seem to do everything slowly.

MY SIMPLE PLAN SIMPLIFIED

Change over gradually to this prudent way of eating, so that eventually you are using healthy ingredients and recipes almost all of the time. You are allowed occasional indulgences of course. Perhaps like me you often fancy a traditional English breakfast at the weekend, or chips may be your particular weakness. If your normal diet is a prudent diet, the odd lapse will not do you any harm. Certainly don't feel guilty about a rare indulgence. You will find after a while that vast meals rich in saturated fats will seem nauseating. You will then have arrived, gently and painlessly, at your diet-of-a-lifetime, which will keep you slim and healthy.

THE TEN FOOD COMMANDMENTS EXPLAINED

1. It is vital to *avoid those fashionable crash diets*. Over 90% of people who try them, revert to their original weight, or eventually get even fatter. Extreme dieting slows down your body's metabolic rate, so that when you return to 'normal' eating the fat soon piles on. Diets also encourage an unhealthy obsession with food. People can become locked into a pattern of denying themselves the calories they need, and then gorging themselves.
2. Eat *far more complex carbohydrates*, including wholemeal bread, flour and pasta, brown rice and potatoes. At the moment 40 to 50% of our typical diet is carbohydrate, but much of it is refined white flour and sugar. Cut those down, while trying to double the quantity of brown bread and potatoes you eat. You should eat at least four slices of wholemeal bread a day, for example, and if that is unavailable, granary and wheatgerm are next best.
3. *Decrease fats to about 30% of your diet* by eating

less fatty meat and dairy products. Meats which are low in fat include chicken, turkey, rabbit, kidney and offal. Try to keep down to one meat meal a day. Cut the fat off meat and choose meals where the meat content is low for about half the time. Two examples are bolognese sauce with pasta and chilli con carne, where the amount of meat is overshadowed by vast quantities of healthy red beans. Increase fish in your diet, while decreasing fried foods drastically. Try using dry skimmed milk for sauces and puddings and silver top or fresh skimmed milk when this is available. Switch to plain yoghurt instead of cream if it makes sense in the recipe. Limit yourself to three eggs a week and reduce intake of fatty cheese. The aim should be to reduce your consumption of saturated fats, so switch from butter to polyunsaturated magarines like Flora and oils like sunflower, safflower and corn oil. Use olive oil, a mono-unsaturate, which is neutral from a health point of view, when it is important for taste. Salad dressings are one example. People who use a lot of olive oil, in areas like the Mediterrean, do not have a high incidence of heart disease and breast cancer. It is the saturated fats which should be avoided.

4. *Less protein is healthy*. At the moment we eat about 12% of protein, but we only need half that amount. It is a good idea to get more protein from grains and vegetables, because these have various health advantages, and less from meat, which often contains a lot of fat.

5. *Reduce salt too*. We now use on average 12 grams per person a day, but ideally we should get that down to six, by using the minimum in cooking and rarely putting it on the table, although it is important for certain recipes, I feel. You can add flavour to food in other ways, especially with spices, herbs and pepper.

6. *Go easy on the sugar*, reducing your consumption by at least 30%, and ideally 50%. We now eat about 100lb each a year, half from the bag and half in pro-

cessed foods. It is easy to use less once you are eating more fresh foods. Tinned fruit, puddings and soft drinks contain alarming quantities. I have eventually learned to prefer tea and coffee without sugar. But I do wish low-calorie drinks did not taste so grim.

7. *Adjust your cooking methods*. Grilling and steaming are far healthier than frying and boiling. You can now buy special pans for fat-free cooking, and woks are ideal for fast-cooking methods which retain crispness and vitamins. A food processor, with its slicing and grating discs makes it simple to add interest to raw vegetables and salad ingredients.

8. *Eat more fresh fruit and vegetables*. Citrus fruits contain flavones while brassicas like sprouts and cauliflower have useful indoles (more about these in my section on Healthy Cooking Methods). Eat dark green vegetables or carrots for vitamins and minerals at least three times a week. Food which is in season and grown locally, ideally in your own garden or allotment, is fresher and cheaper. Increase both fruit and vegetable intake by at least 30%.

9. *Increase fibre* as much as possible, using dried beans, pulses and seeds. It is also contained in fruit, vegetables, cereals and wholemeal bread of course. Some scientists believe that when you eat a lot of fibre, a proportion of the calories are locked up in indigestible roughage which passes quickly through the body. This is one reason why high-fibre food helps you to stay thin.

10. *Eat a wide variety of the foods* recommended above. Don't overcook or overeat. Choose all ingredients which are as fresh as possible — the freezer has a lot to answer for. You will regain an interest in *tasty* food on my Total Health Plan, which you should wash down with a couple of glasses of wine a day or the equivalent. Alcohol in moderation is good for your arteries and it reduces stress.

A DAY IN THE TOTAL HEALTH PLAN

Eating this way should be flexible and extremely varied. But just to help you find your feet, I am outlining a typical day's food. It is important to have three meals, but no snacks, to keep your blood sugar at a fairly constant level.

BREAKFAST is important and, if it has to be missed, make up for it at work or wherever, by taking bread and fruit with you. If you like *high-fibre cereals*, start with these but do not use raw bran. Otherwise have two slices of *wholemeal bread* with a small amount of *polyunsaturated margarine* and home-made or low-sugar jams or marmalade. Always have *fresh fruit*, grapefruit for example, or the juice of two oranges. Tea or coffee should be drunk with *low-fat milk* and *no sugar*.

LUNCH seems to be the ideal time to have raw, fresh vegetables and salads. Eat them with low-fat meats, fish or cottage cheese. Healthy flans, soups and dishes made from dried beans or peas, like hummus, are favourites of mine because I am not a cold salad fan, particularly in the winter. Use bread and potatoes as much as you wish.

DINNER is one of my favourite times of the day because it is the ideal opportunity to relax with the people who most matter with something else that matters to me — good food. And deciding to eat healthy food need not affect the quality of the food, as many traditional health-food fanatics seem to believe. Eat two savoury courses, followed by fresh fruit and/or cheese, with yoghurt for children if they feel they must have some kind of 'pudding'. Eat potatoes in their skins, with large portions of fresh vegetables, lightly cooked in as many different ways as your imagination can devise. Use meat no more than once a day and make it go further with beans and vegetables like aubergines, or in fabulous Italian sauces for pasta. Use a lot of Chinese and Japanese recipes, with little meat and lots of crisp fresh vegetables.

AVOIDING OBESITY WITH THE TOTAL FOOD PLAN

By following this eating plan, you cannot become over-weight and, if you are at the start, you will soon shed pounds. This should happen at a regular but fairly slow pace, with a weight loss of about one or two pounds a week. But, unlike dieting, *this* weight loss will be permanent. By eating less of the calorie-rich sugars and fats and more fibre-rich foods, you will be able to eat more and feel full, without putting on weight. Most of the foods you will eat are bulky and chewy, so you will be able to eat fewer calories without feeling hungry. They also contain lots of water, so that you will often be able to eat ten times as much for the same number of calories. You will feel healthier and reach your ideal weight without any risk of upsetting your body's natural balance, your ideal metabolic rate.

AVOIDING DISEASE WITH THE TOTAL HEALTH PLAN

British medical experts, convinced that 'we are what we eat', are banding together to persuade the Government to invest in more health education about 'eating' and to press for agreements with food suppliers. They are convinced that, as my food plan explains, we should eat less fat, sugar and salt, and move to fibre-rich foods instead. They believe our present, typical diet causes several major diseases, which shorten life and cost the National Health Service up to one billion pounds a year.

The following diseases are linked to our typical Western diet and are rare in other parts of the world where eating patterns are different:

DISEASE	DIETARY CAUSE
Heart Disease	Too much fat
High blood pressure	Too much fat and salt
Obesity	Too much fat, sugar and salt — with too little fibre
Strokes	Too much salt and fat
Diabetes	Too much fat and sugar — too little fibre
Cancer of large bowel and colon, and diverticular disease	Too little fibre
Mineral and vitamin deficiencies	Too much fat, sugar, salt — too little fibre

These ten diseases are often called 'the diseases of civilisation' because we have become progressively more prone to them all as we have become rich enough to move away from simple, fresh, natural foods. A few societies still exist which suffer from none of these problems, including African bushmen, the Kikuyu tribe in Kenya, and the Tarahumura Indians of North Mexico. They eat rough cereals, leaves or roots, no salt and very little meat.

But it has been found that if any members of these tribes move to towns and cities, and alter their diet in the process, they too become prone to those ten diseases which ravage the West. African cities, for example, are becoming full of overweight, middle-class Africans, mirroring the experience in the West over 300 years ago. A visit to the National Portrait Gallery will prove to you that gross obesity was rare until the end of the 17th century, when people began to get richer and so changed their diet.

This discovery by scientists of the amazing health record of primitive tribes, has led to the ultimate irony. Some of the richest and fattest of Americans are now living like the poor Tarahumura tribesmen in one of the richest, most self-indulgent of States — California. At a health centre near Los Angeles, called optimistically the Pritikin LONGEVITY Centre, people are committed enough to their health to pay 6000 dollars over 26 days in the hope of learning a life-style which may earn them a few extra years.

They eat the modern, American equivalent of the simple tribal meal, which is basically lots of fresh fruit, raw vegetables and fibre-rich foods. They exercise under medical supervision, and attend lectures and cookery classes which teach them how to continue this lifestyle at home. When I visited the Longevity Centre myself (not as an inmate I must add) I realised that many people there were frightened by age or ill-health into changing their eating and exercise habits. But some, who seemed young and vibrant, believed in prevention. One lithe and beautiful woman in her late twenties told me she was horrifed by the diet of salty, sugary snacks, fatty fast-foods and fizzy drinks that her five-year-old daughter and her friends lived on in the Texas of today. She said she was learning good habits at the Longevity Centre to pass on to the next generation. She is right of course, but why she needs to spend so much money and time to learn the health message I am not sure.

She certainly should be worried about the effect of fast-foods on the long-term health of her daughter. Hamburgers are a way of life in America, and it is getting that way in Britain too. Even in Japan, where most people eat an extremely healthy diet, and where the average life-expectancy far exceeds ours in the West, a few hamburger chains have appeared. The queues outside are made up largely of obese children, the first generation to be overweight in Japan.

Let me just explain what happens when you eat a standard hamburger, full of fat in the meat, sauce and cheese, with sugary ketchup and a white flour bun. Your blood sugar will quickly rise, your pancreas will

24

push out insulin to cope with that sugar, and then the blood sugar will drop rapidly. Your adrenal glands will pump out adrenaline, which takes starch from the liver and so puts your blood sugar right back up again. The importance of avoiding these fluctuations in blood sugar, both for diabetics and healthy people, is explained in the later section on fibre.

I have yet to meet a child who can resist hamburgers, sold over the counter or made at home. But this is one area for moderation — please!

THE TOTAL FOOD PLAN EXPLAINED

Live and Let Diet
My first of the ten food commandments is to avoid dieting as we know it. Unfortunately diet is a word that has been misinterpreted. It is not just for people who want to slim, it is for us all. Diet means simply *what we eat*, and getting our diet right is one of our two main health challenges.

We've certainly been getting it wrong for years. Diet, to most people, means losing weight put on by eating too many of the wrong foods. Over 60% of us attempt to lose a few of those extra pounds every year. Only 5% sustain that weight loss, so we blame ourselves and feel guilty.

But, in fact, it is the crash diets, and the so-called experts who dream up each weight-reducing gimmick, who should be blamed. Just think how many unscientific and unhealthy diets people have swallowed in recent years. Remember the grapefruit, which was said to shed pounds, then the banana, the orange, and various high-protein regimes? Recently Judy Mazel, with her Beverly Hills Diet, became a millionairess by becoming the pineapple's best friend. The pineapple may be more glam than bran but some scientists have claimed that this diet could be dangerous.

New diets, promoted with great showmanship,

continue to make their authors pounds by falsely promising to help readers lose unwanted pounds. Diets don't produce permanent weight-loss because they are unscientific, but books on the subject continue to sell. Diets are myths which are swallowed by unsuspecting seekers of solutions. People believe that they will not only lose weight, but that once slimmer, they will become happier and more loved. For this reason diets are addictive. And for this reason it will not be easy to persuade people to give them up and to eat healthily instead.

The quest for thin bodies has done a lot of people a lot of harm. Whoever dreamed up that famous quote: 'a woman can never be too thin or too rich' has a lot to answer for. One in every 220 girls in Britain now suffers from anorexia. Many of them are teenagers, hoping for jobs as models or dancers. It starts as an urge to slim, but gets out of hand. 2% of all women in Britain are also thought to suffer from bulima, a condition which involves overeating followed by induced vomiting. These diseases are obviously the most extreme effects of that compulsive urge to be thin, but dieting makes everyone feel bad in some way. When your blood sugars become low you can become very irritable, while the never-ending thought of food makes people introverted and stressed. Surely the time has come to accept that the war against our bodies has had too many casualties, that the war is a wasted war because there is no victory, and that we should now decide that it is time for a truce.

The best way to get slim and stay slim is to throw away all your diet books, and forget about crash diets. The slim-line secret is to eat healthily, without denying yourself, to exercise moderately, and to watch yourself return to your ideal weight, losing at least one or two pounds a week without really trying. And the real slim-line tonic, is that you won't put this weight back on again. It's that simple. It's the diet of a lifetime.

Crash dieting, on the other hand, usually results in you putting on even more weight when you begin to start eating normally again. This is because diets slow down our natural metabolic rate, which is 'the sum total of all the chemical reactions that go on in our living cells'. When our metabolic rate slows down we use less energy. It is quite normal for energy requirements to decrease by 25% during a month of severe dieting.

Once the body's energy needs have been depressed in this way, you put on extra weight when you return to normal eating. And in people who take no exercise, this extra weight is usually in the proportion of more fat than lean tissue. Sedentary people then worry about this weight gain, diet again, eat normally, then diet, and so on, altering the composition of their bodies in an alarming way.

This explains the present situation in Britain, where more of us are getting fatter, although we actually eat fewer calories than a generation ago. It is a frightening contradiction, and the solution can only be found in combining a more active life with healthier eating.

Our generation eats an average of 20 tons of food in a lifetime, and when we get the balance of exercise and food wrong, we put on weight. Many people believe that gaining pounds is an inevitability of middle-age, that it is linked to something mysterious like hormone changes. But this is not so. Weight gain is not inevitable, it is the result of a sedentary life where we get the energy balance wrong. Think of that balance like a seesaw, with the energy input, the food and drink, on one side, and the energy we use up during the day on the other side. Even a small imbalance every day will add up to a huge weight gain over a number of years, and certainly in Britain at the moment the seesaw is heavily weighted down on the side of the energy input.

Energy needs vary enormously from person to person, depending on their physical activity, body weight, metabolic rate and to a lesser extent to age and climate. You can get your personal seesaw in balance by following my exercise and food plans, fitting them into your own particular lifestyle, likes and dislikes. It is an easy way of feeling fitter and happier, while being less prone to several serious diseases.

Eat Double the Quantity of Carbohydrates
This advice may seem an anathema to the traditional dieter. For years people who have wanted to lose weight, as well as those with illnesses like diabetes, have been warned to eat the minimum of carbohydrates. It can be difficult to adjust now that the medical message has changed.

Of course, most of us know that the desirable carbohydrates are unrefined, brown rice, pasta, wholemeal breads, flours and so on. We must still cut down on the refined carbohydrates like white sugar and flour. Only complex, unrefined carbohydrates are desirable for healthy, desirable bodies. One excellent, complex carbohydrate food, for example, is the potato. It contains less than 1% of fat in its natural form. But we have got to lose our fondness for adding fat to our potatoes. Chips contain 80 times more fat than a plain potato, while crisps contain 120 times more. So potatoes should be eaten plain, preferably in their skins where vitamins lurk. The Irish were right, because the potato, like all complex carbohydrates, is the perfect food, providing a constant, slow supply of glucose to the bloodstream. Simple, refined carbohydrates, like sugar and honey, however, flood the system, increasing our chances of suffering from diabetes and hypoglycaemia.

The British Diabetic Association has now endorsed a high carbohydrate/high fibre diet for all patients, which is very different to the old diet for this disease, which restricted carbohydrates. The new diet is the very opposite to our standard British diet of the last thirty years, because starchy, fibrous carbohydrates in the form of beans, cereals, fruit and vegetables, make up 60% of the suggested food.

Starches enter the blood stream more slowly than sugars, and fibre helps to slow the process even more, countering the fluctuations in the important blood sugar level. So the body needs less injected insulin to keep the system in balance. This means a better degree of diabetic control. The new Diabetic diet, which has an accompanying recipe book to encourage patients to make changes, would in fact benefit everyone in Britain, diabetic or not.

Decrease the Fat in Your Diet

Saturated fats are bad for us. Of that there is now no doubt. I will start with heart disease, which has always been controversial as far as fats are concerned. Populations which eat less than 25% of fat rarely suffer from coronary heart disease, and in Japan, where there is only one sixth the amount of CHD as in Britain, people eat very little fat, although they smoke more than us and they do lead stressful lives.

There are definitely several factors involved in the disease, including smoking, lack of exercise, stress and diet. But fats in the diet are particularly significant. They can increase cholesterol levels, which in turn increase the chances of CHD.

Deaths from heart disease more than doubled in England and Wales between 1950 and 1974. In Scotland and Ireland rates are even higher. We are seeing very few improvements here, although the rates have dropped by 20% in America, and improved dramatically in some European countries. There have been various campaigns to persuade people to make lifestyle changes in America, which have been amazingly successful. There has been a reduction in the use of saturated fats, with a move from butter to polyunsaturates and low-fat spreads.

It is becoming easier for people in Britain to make changes because our shops are beginning to sell healthier foods and ingredients. At the back of the book I include lists of supermarkets and other stores, and the efforts they make towards their customers' health. It is certainly easier now to buy polyunsaturated oils like sunflower oil, corn oil and safflower oil. Supermarkets sell their own brands of polyunsaturated and low-fat spreads, which are cheaper than the well-known brands like Flora, Gold and Outline. Scientists have recently discovered that substances contained in polyunsaturated fats help the platelets in our blood, which cause it to clot, to be less sticky. They therefore believe that we should eat more of these to avoid the risk of blood clots. So unless you are severely overweight, they advise polyunsaturated products like Flora, instead of low-fat spreads like Gold and Outline. But obviously no one should eat too many fats of any kind.

Skimmed milk is also recommended by scientists but I do find it difficult to get it fresh and the stuff that is delivered to my door goes off very quickly and has a distinctive metallic taste. I have reluctantly gone back to silver top. It is also wise to reduce meat meals to one a day, to cut the fat off meat, to use low-fat cheeses and yoghurt, and to remember not to go to work on an egg. Three a week is quite enough.

The US National Academy of Sciences report, 1982, on the relationship between diet and cancer, concluded that fat in the diet should be reduced to 30%, because high levels increased the risk of cancer of the breast and colon. Some studies suggest that fat encourages the secretion of bile steroids and acids which might encourage tumours.

Should we shake the Salt Habit?

The debate over salt has been going on for centuries. The Chinese emperor Huang Ti said, as long ago as the 27th century BC: 'if too much salt is used in food, the pulse hardens.' But we love salt, and in fact, when it first became cheap enough to add to every pan and every table, we soon increased our intake ten times. As the old Sanskrit proverb says; 'There are six flavours and of them all salt is the greatest.'

But today many scientists do not share that enthusiasm because they believe that using a lot of salt can cause medical problems. The discussion paper on *Proposals for Nutritional Guidelines for Health Education in Britain*, published in the autumn of 1983, advised reducing salt intake. It explained that: 'Animal experiments have shown that very high intakes of sodium lead to high levels of blood pressure and that modest intakes of sodium can lead to hypertension [high blood pressure] in genetically susceptible animals.' It also mentioned human experiments which showed that low-salt diets could lower blood pressure, and concluded; 'The present estimated average intake of salt in Britain amounts to 12g per day if allowances are made for additions made in cooking and at table. . . . A salt intake of 12g a day is far in excess of that required even by physically active individuals and a gradual reduction to a half or even a quarter of this level is unlikely to be associated with any danger to health.'

Our bodies do need a certain amount of sodium from salt (sodium chloride). It is involved in vital functions, including nerve impulses and heart action and we have methods of conserving sodium in both urine and sweat. But some scientists now believe that most of us use at least twice the amount of salt that we need to be healthy. They are still not sure if saltaholic behaviour leads to health problems for all of us, but there is a lot of epidemiological evidence to suggest that salt can cause high blood pressure and strokes. In Japan, for example, where a lot of salt is used in pickles and soya sauce, many people do die from strokes. In some villages, at least 40% of the population have high blood pressure.

So although the scientific arguments for and against salt have not yet been fully resolved, it does seem sensible to use it sparingly. Salt substitutes are now on sale in Britain, although it could be easier just to get used to eating food with less salt. The taste for salt quickly disappears for most people, and in excess it dulls the taste buds. There are so many other flavourings we can use instead, including garlic, cumin, vinegar, angostura bitters, tabasco, peppers and lemon. After using them with imagination, salt can soon become just a memory.

But you also have to know where salt is found in food, to be sure that you can avoid it. Only 5 to 10% is found naturally in food, mostly in meat, we tend to add between 20 and 40% during cooking or at the table, and between 30 and 70% is in processed food. That level is alarmingly high, but although salt was removed from baby foods after pressure from the public, very little is being done to reduce levels in other processed foods.

The advantage of my Total Health Plan, however, is that most of the foods are fresh. You go a long way towards reducing the quantity of salt eaten, by eliminating most of the processed foods from your diet. I also only put salt on the table rarely, when the food really demands it. I use salt sparingly in cooking. My family are certainly not feeling the pinch, or lack of it, and after just a few weeks of eating less salt I am sure that you will feel the same. Beware of salty foods like Worcestershire and Soya sauces, cured meat and fish, stock cubes, chutneys and tomato ketchup. Use them carefully.

Although I now believe that salt is over-rated, I would never ask keen cooks, if they could manage without it altogether. If I did, I would expect them to reply saltily in the negative. But I do believe that we abuse the salt cellar at the moment, and could all do well by remembering what happens in one famous restaurant if customers shake salt on their food without tasting it first. They are shaken out of the restaurant, never to return. And quite right too.

HEALTHY COOKING METHODS

We ought to give some thought to the way we cook food. Our reputation for over-boiled, soggy cabbage and limp, fatty chips is well-deserved. For the past year I have been gradually making changes and we have never enjoyed our food more. For a start I bought a second wok.

WOKS are common in China and many other countries in the Far-East and you can now find them in almost every British High Street. They are extremely versatile, coping with braising, steaming and casseroling, as well as normal quick frying. They originated in China about 2000 years ago and were used over open fires, where the flat bottom allowed a lot of food to come into contact with the heat. *Quick stir-frying* is popular in the wok, where small, evenly-sized pieces of vegetable, fish or meat are constantly stirred while being cooked for only a few minutes. In this way, the food keeps its colour, consistency, vitamins and other nutrients. Another advantage is that very, very little oil (polyunsaturated of course) is needed and any excess will drain back into the centre. This is definitely one of the healthiest, tastiest and most nutritious methods of cooking. *Steaming* is another excellent way of making use of the wok. Fish, especially, is perfect cooked in this way. Place it on a steam rack, over a few tablespoons of water, sprinkle with seasoning and finely chopped vegetables. After steaming, the liquid in the base has collected all the juices and goodness. It will make a good accompanying sauce. Certainly don't waste it.

GRILLING is much better than frying for handling more traditional British ingredients like chops, steaks and bacon. Try to avoid the frying pan as we know it. One portion of grilled bacon, for example, saves 100 calories compared to the same portion fried.

BAKING AT LOW TEMPERATURES has several advantages. If you put food like potatoes, vegetables and fruit in a cold oven and heat up slowly, they will retain their vitamins and minerals. The oven should be set at about 300 F (Gas no 2), but when the food is completely heated through, which is when it is steaming and bubbling, turn the oven down to 200 F (Gas no ¼) to finish cooking. This prevents skins becoming tough while keeping the flavour excellent.

STEAMING, using a traditional saucepan with a steamer inside, is preferable to boiling because the food does not come into direct contact with the boiling water so that more of its flavour and nutrients are retained.

VACUUM COOKING, MICROWAVE COOKING AND SPECIAL PANS FOR FAT-FREE COOKING have all been recommended to me, although I have not tried them myself. But I do advocate the use of brushes to mop fat from the surface of sauces and I own a sauce boat where the funnel begins at the bottom of the dish so any fat is left behind.

FIBRE

INCREASE FIBRE, including beans and pulses, and eat at least one third more fresh FRUIT and VEGETABLES. Fibre has had such a good press recently that there doesn't seem to be much more to say about it. Although one fact may have escaped you. Did you know it has become *so* fashionable that even hens have now been put on high-fibre diets? In America of course. The idea is to reduce the amount of cholesterol in eggs. It could only happen in America.

But ignoring that, let me summarize the known advantages of high fibre in the human diet. It helps you to slim, because by the time you feel full from the bulky, chewy food you will still not have consumed many calories. Some fibre foods reduce the dangerous cholesterol in your blood, and all are ideal for diabetics, improving glucose tolerance. Fibre protects against bowel problems by increasing the weight of the faeces and shortening food transit time. The concentration of cancer-inducing contents in the bowel are thought to be reduced by the fatty acids produced when fibre is digested.

Before we leave fibre, there are a few drawbacks to report. Flatulence is one of them — most people know that to their cost. Also, the surprising news from scientists that raw bran is not perfect after all. There is phytic acid in raw bran that can interfere with the absorption of calcium, magnesium, iron and zinc, which can be a particular problem if you are pregnant or elderly. Try breakfast cereals like porridge, which are based on oats, for a change. They certainly make horses lively. Get most of your fibre from wholemeal bread. We can live without raw bran. After all fibre turns up in plenty of other sources — some very unlikely places indeed, even in beer, like stout. So it could be true what they say about Guinness!

Vegetables and fruit are extremely important too. One study has suggested that vegetarians live longer than average, as well as suffering from far less high blood pressure than most people. This is thought to be due to the protective effect of potassium, which is high in a vegetable-rich diet. It is also believed by some scientists that vegetables from the brassica family, like turnips, cauliflower, sprouts and so on, contain organic chemicals called indoles which cause enzymes to be formed which protect against cancer. Citrus fruits are thought to contain flavones, and beans and seeds lectins, which also protect against cancer.

THE ROYAL COLLEGE OF PHYSICIANS 'OBESITY' REPORT

When this report was published last year, we were all alarmed to learn that 40% of British men and over 30% of British women are now overweight. The report urged us to change to the sort of diet I have just recommended, low in fat and sugar, and high in starchy, fibrous carbohydrates. That is something we can do ourselves. But we can only wait and hope that the Royal College of Physicians gets its way in insisting that packaged foods are labelled for nutrient and calorie content, and that Government and Industry get together over a new Code of Practice. The report claims, for example, that Government policies encouraging dairy and meat, instead of cereal farming, are wrong.

Those sort of changes will take time. What we need from the Government now, is some effective way of getting the message about healthy eating over to everyone, especially those who most need it. One of the most alarming aspects of the increase in obesity, and diseases like coronary heart disease, is that poorer people are now becoming more susceptible. Until the 1950's, heart disease was a rich man's problem, caused by high living. But now the disease is affecting more poor families, who are becoming overweight, and are suffering from the 'diseases of civilisation', because they are, increasingly, eating the WRONG type of calories. They eat 56% less fruit, 19% less fresh vegetables and 32% more sugar than families higher up the social scale.

School meals and other institutional food, repeat these mistakes. A survey of Royal Navy personnel showed that 28% of them were obese, despite their active life. When the kitchens were examined, it was seen that fresh fruit and wholemeal bread were rare. Vegetables were so overcooked, that few vitamins would escape the attack.

Many health experts worry that an inadequate diet can be blamed on low incomes rather than lack of knowledge. But, having worked out my food plan and lived with it for a year, I know that it is cheaper than the average British diet. Vegetables and bread are cheaper than fatty meats and creamy puddings. Supermarket chains now sell brown rice and wholemeal pasta as cheaply as their refined versions. I am quite sure that we can all, whatever our income, stop the rot and live longer, livelier lives.

SUGAR

We still need to go easy on the sugar, although this is one of the few 'food' areas where we can boast improvements. Our consumption of sugar is down by one third over the last ten years, but it is still far too high. Britain uses more sugar per head than anywhere else in the world. We eat on average 4 oz of refined sugar each a day, which provides 450 cals — over one quarter of our average daily calorie needs. One extra problem is that those calories are empty calories, because sugar contains nothing valuable like vitamins.

We need to reduce the amount of sugar we use by at least a third, as one to two ounces a day would be far more realistic. Sugar is still causing us problems in Britain. It has been blamed for many problems from obesity, to coronary heart disease, diabetes, kidney damage and perhaps breast cancer. In trying to cut down, we not only have to watch the amount of loose sugar we use, but we have to remember that many processed foods are full of it. Tomato ketchup, for example, contains 20%. Even the so-called 'goodies' can be a problem. Some muesli is one quarter sugar, fruit yoghurt often contains about 18%, and many bran-based breakfast cereals are at least 15% sugar.

POSTSCRIPT

— or my last word on the Total Food Plan

It has often been said that books are read by the middle-classes, and especially by women. So how can I hope that my message gets passed on to everyone who needs it? Well, apart from finding that my friends and relatives are incredibly eager to know the secrets of food health, I am passing on the knowledge I have gained to my children every day.

Most young children get enough exercise of course, so we don't have to worry about that. But, what with school lunches, tuck shops and sweet counters at the station where they go off to school, their eating habits can become very unhealthy. It is possible, however, to fire their enthusiasm for changes. Although my two sons, Jake, aged fourteen, and Daniel, now twelve, groaned when the chip pan was first banned, they now realise that they are able to have deep-fried food when they go out to friends, restaurants and so on. And they now enjoy chips even more, because they are a rare treat.

They were instantly enthusiastic about brown rice and wholemeal bread and pasta. They have already lost their sweet and salt cravings. Fresh fruit and yoghurts are preferred to sticky puddings. Also, when they moaned about school dinners and I discovered how grim they were, I grabbed at the opportunity of changing them over from those bad, institutional offerings, to much fresher, healthier packed lunches. As a guide to any other parents who want to do this, they have hot vegetable soups in the winter, and throughout the year they have wholemeal bread, spread with a thin layer of polyunsaturated margarine. The fillings vary between salads, vegetables, fish or low-fat meats. They take fresh fruit or yoghurt, with fresh fruit drinks.

I am sure that it is easier to alter eating preferences

in childhood rather than later. And the sooner the changes are made, the greater the chances of avoiding the 'diseases of civilisation' which shorten and disfigure life.

3   The Total Exercise Plan

THE TEN EXERCISE COMMANDMENTS

1. Never take exercise to extremes.

2. Just one hour of exercise a week keeps you fit.

3. Consider your body type.

4. Always exercise aerobically.

5. Be aware of the disadvantages of anaerobic exercise.

6. Decide on exercise that you really enjoy.

7. Gradually build up the intensity of the exercise during each session.

8. Change the type of exercise you do from time to time.

9. Take care when first exercising after years of inactivity.

10. Remember the importance of warming-up and cooling-down periods.

If I had to single out the most significant mistake we are making in health terms, it would be our lack of exercise. Britain is a nation of fatties, and the most alarming aspect of this trend towards obesity, is that we are getting fatter despite eating fewer calories than we did a generation ago.

The main reason for this is that most of us now lead sedentary lives, and when we are inactive our energy balance goes wrong. If the energy input, from food and drink, outweighs the energy used up in general activity and exercise, we become fat. The Royal College of Physicians 1983 report on *Obesity* urged that 'All adults should remain physically active throughout life.' It claimed that it was vital for our health that we should change our attitude to exercise.

Of course lack of exercise does not just lead to obesity. It is thought to increase our chances of suffering from several diseases, including heart disease, which shorten our lives. Scientists at the London School of Hygiene and Tropical Medicine discovered that men working as conductors on London's double-decker buses suffered from only half as many heart attacks as the bus drivers. They then found that postmen had similar advantages over Government clerks. Although it is possible that the more active jobs attracted fitter, healthier people, it is also likely that the conductors and the postmen were less prone to heart disease because they did not lead sedentary lives. Certainly there was far less heart disease in the days before motor transport, television and desk-bound work.

The answer today is to make up for our sedentary lifestyle by taking exercise. A survey of 18,000 British civil servants found that those who took exercise in their leisure time were far less likely to suffer from heart disease. Another major study, in Baltimore, USA, has also concluded that exercise is effective in keeping us healthier and younger. The Gerontology Centre in Baltimore is studying thousands of people as they age. The same patients return for testing at regular intervals throughout their lives, and the aim of the study is to understand how we all age. One major conclusion of the scientists is that exercise has many benefits.

It has been found, from several studies, that people who continue to exercise or lead very active lives, into old age, have a lower 'functional' age than actual years. One study showed that those who exercise regularly live on average seven years longer than sedentary people.

But exercise must never be taken to extremes. Experts recommend about 20 minutes of MODERATE activity three times a week. They say this is enough to make you healthier, benefiting the heart, lungs and circulation. They believe that Britain is so far behind other countries in realising the need for a healthy lifestyle, with this type of moderate exercise, that they are demanding a major health promotion campaign.

Such campaigns have been effective in America, reducing the heart disease rate dramatically. Canada has also carried out an imaginative national fitness survey, on an age-range from seven to seventy. They have collected data on exercise behaviour and attitudes, as well as measuring fitness, muscular strength, flexibility and body composition. The *British Medical Journal* stated recently that: 'Such a national fitness survey is now being considered for Britain; the interest and enthusiasm for sport and exercise it could be expected to generate, the new information it would yield on the people's health, and its baseline for monitoring progress could well add a new dimension to the national effort in health promotion and health education.'

We are still way behind many other countries in our attitude to exercise, but fortunately more British people are beginning to realise the importance of swimming, cycling, aerobic dancing, walking and moderate jogging. A year ago a scientific symposium on exercise and health was sponsored by the Medical Research Council, Health Education Council and the Sports Council. Their conclusions are filtering through to doctors, and gradually to the general public. It has been said that the use of exercise for improving health, is in a state of transition from unfounded faddism to scientific legitimacy. That transition needs to be speeded up in Britain by more scientific meetings and more effective public health campaigns. Then the number of people taking exercise should increase dramatically, and the British public could then be said — literally — to be voting with its feet.

THE TOTAL EXERCISE PLAN EXPLAINED

Just a small amount of the sort of aerobic exercise you enjoy, can have a massive effect on your health, making you feel better mentally as well as increasing your fitness.

Never Take Exercise to Extremes
Exercise has had a very bad Press recently. Anti-jogging lobbies and worried doctors have been warning us of the risks of heart attacks, fractures, concussion, torn ligaments, cauliflower ears and even jogger's nipple. It seems that exercise can be so addictive, that many people are taking it to extremes. Doctors even have a term for the damage suffered by obsessive exercisers. They call it 'self-abuse'.

The worst examples of self-abuse are found amongst the long-distance joggers and the addicts of rough, tough sports. It seems that many people who begin as gentle joggers end up, like lemmings, running marathon after marathon. And while this may be sensible for the very fit or young, it is not a good idea for most of us. In San Francisco people are so keen on this form of exercise that they go to classes to learn 'how to jog'. But a study done in the city concluded that more than half of all sudden deaths from coronary heart disease occurred during or just after strenuous exercise. And a team from the University of Auckland, New Zealand, discovered that an alarming number of people dying suddenly, had recently taken up running as a form of exercise. None of the patients had complained of cardiac symptoms during the day before their death, but all had historical evidence of abnormal coronary disease risk factors. The scientists suggest that they should have been diagnosed by their doctors as being at risk, and encouraged to take less strenuous forms of exercise.

It is an unfortunate dilemma that patients with coronary heart disease, who are at greatest risk of exercise-related problems and sudden death, may also benefit from exercise. The scientists recommend that doctors be aware of the potential dangers of excessive exercise for all their patients. And with heart disease patients in particular, moderate physical activity like swimming or brisk walking is advised.

These two studies are obviously extreme examples of the dangers of excessive exercise. But there are lessons we can all learn from them. If you have mild high blood pressure, if you have ever suffered from heart problems like angina, or if you are overweight, talk to your doctors before taking exercise. It is almost certain that you can benefit from exercise. But moderation, which is important for all of us, is particularly important for you.

There are several common problems that can occur if you exercise to excess. A friend said to me the other day: 'What sort of exercise should my husband take in between his running?' I was puzzled by this odd question, until she told me that he suffers from regular knee and ankle joint problems, and could only run on his odd 'good days'. Although both she and her husband blame bad running shoes, which can obviously cause problems, I told her that it was far more likely to be the running itself. His body was telling him that running was unsuitable for him. I advised more gentle aerobic exercise, and I expect his aches and pains to end.

One study done by the Centre for Disease Control in Atlanta, America, on 1,500 runners, found that one third of them averaging more than six miles a week, suffer from injuries to knees, ankles and other joints within one year of starting this strenuous exercise. Half of them were bad enough to need medical attention.

Long distance running is also known to damage muscles, body cells and even the kidneys in extreme cases. Child runners can suffer from stunted growth, and back disorders are also common. Women may become so thin after taking extreme exercise every day that they suffer from menstrual disfunction. In fact, scientists believe that if body fat drops below 17% of a woman's total weight she is at risk of becoming infertile. There are many cases of women runners suffering from infertility and hormonal changes. The only answer is to take it easy. We all need exercise. But, ironically, we can damage ourselves by trying too hard to do ourselves good.

Psychologists at the University of Arizona believe that people obsessed with running to keep fit may be afflicted in the same way as women with anorexia. A study of 60 marathon runners found they had similar personality traits to anorexics, particularly introversion and the inability to express anger. The runners drove themselves to get fitter but no goal was ever good enough, just as anorexics think they are still fat, even when they have become dangerously thin. Compulsive runners and anorexics strive to establish a more stable identity through their extreme behaviour.

Just One Hour of Exercise A Week Keeps You Fit
Sixty minutes of exercise a week does not sound very

much. But if it is the right kind of exercise done in the correct way, it will keep you fit and happy. The Royal College of Physicians Report on *Obesity* recommended 20 minutes of moderate activity three times a week. The experts who compiled the report are convinced that one hour a week is enough to 'maintain cardiovascular reflex responses to physical activity'. In other words it will maintain your heart and blood supply in a healthy state.

It has also been found that by keeping up this one hour of moderate exercise over a period of time, people can lower their blood pressure levels. The normal decline with age of bone mineral density is also delayed by exercise. This is particularly good news for elderly women who are more at risk from brittle bones. Regular, moderate exercise could protect them from this problem of old age.

Exercise will also help anyone who is overweight. The types of exercise I recommend speed up the body's metabolic rate, and help you to lose weight. My exercise plan will leave you slimmer, fitter, healthier and happier.

The evidence for my last claim, that exercise makes you feel better, is interesting. Scientists found that many people taking regular exercise claimed to have an increased tolerance to pain, a reduction in stress, and a feeling of euphoria. Research provided the explanation. Blood samples were taken during exercise, and it was discovered that unusually high quantities of a natural opiate were present. This is a hormone produced by the brain and pituitary gland, called beta-endorphin, which makes you feel good and happy. Scientists now believe that exercise can become addictive to some people, just because this hormone makes them feel euphoric.

There is a second advantage in exercising to produce beta-endorphin. It has been found that there are special receptors on our lymphocytes (the body cells which fight disease) for beta-endorphin, and experiments have shown that this natural opiate makes lymphocytes over 20% more effective at warding off infections. This might explain why people who exercise regularly seem to avoid illness.

If exercise really does prevent disease and lengthen life, then the fitness craze could become the largest long-term study in medical history!

Consider Your Body Type
You probably heard about 'body types' at school, although it is hardly the kind of subject that comes up later in life — in the office or at the pub. But just as a reminder — there are three basic body types.

THE ENDOMORPH tends to be short and fat. If you are this type you probably had to put up with your games teacher insisting that you would be no good for the athletics team, and a disaster at long-distance running. He might have suggested that you train as a weight lifter.

THE MESOMORPH is muscular and fairly lean. This type was always popular for most school sports, particularly running and pole vaulting. But all sports and exercise are easy.

THE ECTOMORPH is a little too tall and too thin to shine on the sports field, except perhaps at high-jump. But the social sports, which we are more likely to carry on past our school years, like tennis, badminton and swimming are no problem for this body type.

Fortunately the types of exercise I recommend, like cycling, swimming and brisk walking, can be enjoyed by endomorphs, mesomorphs and ectomorphs alike. They keep you healthy regardless of shape and body size, they exercise most parts of the anatomy, and they put very little strain on the body. But many people reading my Total Health Plan will want to get their weekly hour of exercise by taking part in sports and games rather than gentle exercise, because they enjoy the social side of playing tennis or whatever. They need to remember that it is important to choose a sport that is right for their body type, and to play that sport in a healthy way. The healthy way is AEROBICALLY, which I explain in the next section.

Always Exercise Aerobically
This is the most important exercise advice of all, because it is aerobic exercise that leads to total health. So what is it? Well it is probably most simply explained as steady, fairly vigorous exercise, which is done at a constant pace, working up a sweat for at least 12 minutes of your three weekly 20-minute exercise sessions.

The vital word is STEADY, because once exercise becomes too intense it is no longer aerobic. When you are exercising aerobically, you are using a sustained supply of oxygen, breathed in from the air. By following my exercise plan you will increase the amount of oxygen your body uses, which will benefit your lungs, heart, blood vessels and your figure.

There are three other types of exercise, which are not so beneficial. At the best they will make your fitter. But they will not improve your health in the same way as aerobic exercise.

ISOMETRICS are exercises which strengthen muscles by tensing them against themselves or an immovable object. They have the disadvantage of pushing up the blood pressure and slowing the flow of blood back to the heart. They involve the type of effort used in straining to lift an impossibly heavy load, pulling on a corkscrew when the cork will not shift, or attempting to push a car up a hill. Isometrics may strengthen your muscles, but they might be bad for your heart, back and temper.

ISOTONICS are exercises where the muscles are free to move because the load on them is only moderate or light. The tension in the muscles stays about the same throughout the exercises, and the muscles are strengthened while the body is exercised in general. Weight training, PT at school, and many of the standard exercises recommended for doing at home, fall into this category. But isotonics, although useful in their own way, do not necessarily increase the amount of oxygen used by the body, unless they are done with steady breathing. So they normally only improve fitness, and do not strengthen your lungs and heart.

ANAEROBIC SPORTS are not steady. They are erratic and often intense, and include the competitive sports like squash and basketball, which involve sudden sprints or bursts of activity. At these times the body cannot get all the oxygen it needs, so you can become extremely breathless. Far from being healthy, anaerobic exercise can be dangerous if you are unfit, as I will explain later.

AEROBIC exercise can be more relaxed, and far more fun, because it is steadier and easier than anaerobic exercise. Choose from the following list, depending on your interests and skills:

SWIMMING is an excellent aerobic exercise because though you use most parts of your body, you don't end up feeling sweaty and uncomfortable. It is easy for most swimmers to keep up a good, vigorous, steady pace for 20 minutes.

CYCLING is another good choice, particularly for people who can fit it easily into their lifestyle by cycling to work or to the local shops. It is necessary, of course, to keep up a steady, and fairly hard pace.

BRISK WALKING is easy to keep up until old age. Walk your dog, enjoy the countryside, or walk through town to work instead of sitting in traffic jams. And finish off this convenient form of aerobic exercise by using the stairs in all buildings you visit, instead of lifts.

AEROBIC DANCE is increasingly popular, especially with younger women. Most people pay to join in group

49

sessions, but this does demand time and sociability. So, for those of you who prefer to exercise in private, at no cost, I include a personal aerobic exercise routine at the back of this book. You will need to choose music with a regular beat to exercise to. Be vigorous, but keep it steady.

DISCO DANCING, CANOEING, DIGGING THE GARDEN, ROWING and even SEX are all good aerobic exercises if kept up at a steady pace for 20 minutes. So you have a big and interesting choice!

TENNIS, BADMINTON and certain other sports can be aerobic if played at a good, steady pace. If you have some skill it is more likely that you will keep running. But if you are so bad at these sports that you spend half the time racing and half the time standing still, they will not improve your health.

JOGGING, or gentle running, is of course aerobic and cheap. But it will not do you any good if you take it to extremes and run long distances every day. Remember the loneliness of the long distance runner — and beware of hard pavements and exhaust fumes. Gentle running, cycling and brisk walking, are all more relaxing and relevant in the country. I think there are better forms of exercise, like swimming and aerobic dance, for towns and cities.

The important thing is to get the balance right. If your way of life is active, with plenty of walking or gardening, you will need to take less organised exercise. And you must plan your aerobic exercise to suit your own age, fitness and health, remembering that when you exercise it is important to raise your heart rate past a certain point, to between 60 and 80% of its maximum.

The most accurate way of checking if you are exercising aerobically is to take your pulse rate. This is quite easy to do. Assuming you are wearing your watch, with a second hand, on your left wrist, take the tips of your fingers of the left hand and put them on the inside of your right wrist near the base of the thumb. You should find your pulse with no difficulty. Count the beats for six seconds on your watch, and then multiply by ten to get your rate per minute. The best time to take the pulse rate is immediately after your normal exercise session.

Your pulse rate will tell you if you are getting the pace of the exercise right. If it is too gentle, and your pulse rate is less than 60% of its maximum, you are not exercising aerobically. If your pulse rate is too high, it can be dangerous. One important thing to remember is that maximum heart rates vary with age, from about 200 beats per minute in the early twenties, to around 150 when you are over sixty. As you become fitter and healthier, you will find that you can do more exercise at a lower pulse rate. But if you are beginning to take exercise for the first time in many years, take it easy and rest if necessary between exercises to keep the pulse rate safely low.

If you do not want to bother with taking your pulse rate because you know you are fairly fit, there is another, simpler way of telling if you are exercising aerobically. It is sometimes known as the 'talk test'. If you are so breathless and exhausted that you cannot talk to a companion during exercise then you are pushing yourself too hard, your pulse rate is too high, and you are in oxygen debt.

AEROBIC ADVANTAGES soon become obvious once you have mastered this form of steady, pleasurable exercise. Your blood vessels will become more elastic, your heart will be stronger, and both your resting heart rate and your blood pressure can drop substantially. Your skin should also improve as new, small blood vessels develop, which encourage new skin growth. Scientists also have evidence that aerobic exercise slows down the tendency for bone to become brittle with age. This is one reason why it is so impor-

51

tant for more elderly people to take exercise. Many of the older scientists working in this field are regular swimmers and cyclists.

The other good news about aerobics is that these exercises help you to lose weight. Within a year of following my Total Health Plan, and taking only one hour of exercise a week, I had shed over a stone and was back to my 'ideal' and most suitable weight of 10 stone.

To explain why aerobic exercise helps to shed weight I need to explain about the two types of muscle fibre we have in our bodies. One form of fibre, called the slow-twitch muscle fibre, is used during aerobic exercise. The fast-twitch fibre, used for work needing immediate reaction, is important in anaerobic exercise. These two different types of muscle fibre use different kinds of fuel to produce energy. And the reason why aerobic exercise helps you to lose weight is that slow-twitch muscle fibres use fat from our body's stores in liquid form as their fuel. Fast-twitch fibres, on the other hand, use glycogen to provide energy. Any weight loss is glycogen plus water bound up with it, which is quickly replaced after exercise. That is why anaerobic exercise does not help you to lose body fat. It cannot reduce your weight permanently. The other bad news about fast-twitch fibres is that if you lead a sedentary life you are likely to have more of them. Slow-twitch can degenerate into fast-twitch if you do not exercise. So you gradually lose the ability to lose fat. You have been warned.

Be Aware of the Disadvantages of Anaerobic Exercise

I have already explained some of the problems of anaerobic exercise, especially its links with fast-twitch fibres and its inability to help you lose weight. But if you are determined to play sports like squash, hockey, football, basketball or karate, there are ways of reducing the problems they can cause. Try to play these games at a steady pace. It is erratic, sudden, fast sprints that should be avoided.

During sudden fast exercise, like sprinting, the demands for energy by the working muscles cannot be met quickly enough by aerobic energy metabolism, so anaerobic pathways must be used. The muscle converts glycogen to lactate, which provides a small amount of energy very quickly. But an increase in lactate concentration has a detrimental effect on muscle. It leads to fatigue.

Unlike aerobic exercise, anaerobic activity can produce dramatic alterations in blood flow. This can be explained by understanding how the muscles learn to need less blood after regular aerobic exercise. The aerobic ability of our muscles is improved by regular, steady exercise, which means they can extract oxygen from the blood more effectively, and therefore tolerate a lower blood flow. So the direct benefit of aerobic exercise is that, with the muscles needing less, blood can be redistributed to the gut, kidneys and liver. Our body does not have to undergo such dramatic changes in blood flow as it does during anaerobic exercise. It has been found that these changes can dislodge plaques, depositing them in coronary arteries and causing an infarction. They can also deplete the heart muscle of its readily available energy source, giving rise to heart attacks.

That is why it is so dangerous for unfit, middle-aged men and women to suddenly take up an anaerobic form of exercise like squash, which claims many lives every year.

Decide on Exercise That You Really Enjoy
The only chance you have of sticking to your Total Exercise Plan is to choose exercise you really enjoy, which fits easily into your present lifestyle. For example, there is no point in a very busy person, who abhors 'body-beautiful' attitudes, joining an expensive health club where most of the other members love

nothing better than to flex their muscles and discuss their weight. To get your moneysworth from this sort of club, you have to be willing and able to use the facilities at least three times a week. Few people with demanding jobs or families can do that.

You will have far more chance of keeping to your plan if you are realistic about exercise from the very beginning. So do give a lot of thought to what is best for you and your lifestyle. For example, do you prefer exercising in a group, so that there are other people to motivate you, and no home or family distractions? If so, aerobic dance classes may be the answer. They are often held in the evenings, although lunch-time sessions are arranged in some towns and cities. You obviously have to have the time, money and inclination. This is not the ideal exercise for anyone who is hard up or shy.

Solitary exercise is the inevitable choice for everyone living too far away from sports facilities, dance classes and health clubs. It is also more realistic for busy people, and for mothers of young children, who do not want the chore of finding baby sitters everytime they need exercise. But if you exercise alone it is essential to be disciplined enough to keep to a regular schedule. After a time, however, your exercise plan should fit naturally into your normal daily routine.

Gradually Build Up the Intensity of the Exercise
Whatever exercise you choose, gradually build up its intensity during each 20-minute session, so that you end up feeling that you have pushed your body and made it work. I have explained the importance of raising the pulse rate, and how to measure it easily. You need to spend at least half of the 20 minutes exercising at a level where your pulse rate is 60% to 80% of its maximum to have a beneficial effect on your body.

You may also find that you want to build up the intensity of your exercise over the weeks and months, to tackle a more ambitious schedule because you are feeling fitter. This is quite natural, but do not be tempted to push yourself too far. I have already talked about the dangers of becoming addicted to exercise, because the brain produces its own natural opiates which make you feel high. Ego also tempts many people to attempt too much. The end result is strained muscles and joints. Remember that the strength of your muscles may be greater than the efficiency of your heart and lungs. So if you do too much, you will end up puffing and panting, with a thumping heart. That is not what aerobic exercise is all about, and it is certainly not good for your body. It is important to keep to a 20-minute session, starting slowly, and building up to your own ideal pulse rate. Then your lungs, heart, blood vessels, figure and state of mind will improve.

Warming-Up and Cooling-Down Periods Are Essential

Although the intensity of exercise should build up during the session, it is important to start slowly, and to allow the body to cool off afterwards. The warm-up period is vital because it allows the heart to increase its rate gradually, while giving the blood vessels a chance to dilate so that they can accommodate the increased blood flow which is inevitable during aerobic exercise. The length of the warm-up period depends on the weather. If it is a warm day and you are fairly fit, five minutes is the perfect time. If it is cold, if you have high blood pressure, or if you are severely unfit, give another five minutes to warming up.

During this time take it very easy, starting slowly and ending with your pulse rate up to the ideal level. I explain warm-up exercises in my aerobic home exercise routine, but if you are choosing other exercises, like swimming, cycling, brisk walking and so on, just begin the session gently, take it easy for five minutes, but end that period by having built up to the ideal exercise intensity. In the same way, end your exercise session by easing off for three or four minutes.

Vary the Exercise You Do From Time to Time
Variety is important, both to avoid monotony and to benefit medically. If you limit yourself to one type of exercise you develop only certain muscle groups, leaving others to stagnate. The importance of getting the total exercise package right was explained to me by RAF staff, who now use a computer to help them find the correct exercise routines for their recruits. In the past, all new recruits were timed during a 12-minute run to check their fitness. But they realised that this gave only a very crude result, because motivation and body type varied from one recruit to another.

Now, measurements of body fat, blood pressure, pulse rates and so on, are fed into the computer along with family medical history, exercise preferences, daily routine and age. The end result is an exercise schedule for each recruit which is far more individual. It suits his health, personality and body type.

When my measurements and personal details were fed into this RAF computer, it was discovered that my Total Exercise Plan, of swimming, walking and a little cycling, had left my heart and lungs in an extremely healthy state. But I had not quite got the total package right. I had spare body fat around the waist area, because I was taking no exercise which firmed up that part of the body. It had never occurred to me before, but apparently even champion runners and swimmers can have badly-toned upper bodies because their form of exercise does not benefit every muscle group.

So I now think about the total effect of the exercise that I do, although I still limit myself to activity which fits easily into my busy lifestyle. For example, I get some basic exercise every morning when I walk my dog. I go on a 20-minute walk with him for his pleasure, but I make sure it is also useful to me by walking briskly most of the time. When I can get out of the city, I also cycle, because my whole family enjoy getting around the countryside on two wheels instead of four. But I would never choose to cycle in a polluted, busy city like London.

I therefore get my 60 minutes of aerobic exercise in London by swimming for two of the sessions a week, and doing aerobic, body-firming exercises at home for the third to get to those parts of my body which swimming can't reach. I made this particular choice because I am not a health club fan, nor a 'group-exerciser'. Swimming is an ideal exercise, because it uses most parts of your body without imposing strain on joints like jogging does. I find that I can think through my day, relax and enjoy myself as I swim up and down in the early morning. I am lucky enough to have a lovely pool near my house, which opens early so that people can exercise before work. If your local pool does not open early enough, get a few people to complain, and it soon will.

After Years of Inactivity Exercise With Care
Many of you may be reading this book because after years of being a slob you have decided to do something about it. You badly need exercise if you experience any of the following:
— You cannot walk briskly and talk to someone at the same time.
— You wake up feeling stiff every morning, and find it difficult to bend and twist throughout the day.
— You find it hard to get to sleep because of tension and over-tiredness.
— The thought of playing tennis or swimming fills you with horror and feelings of fatigue.
— Your naked shape in the mirror makes you feel ashamed.

So you need my Total Exercise Plan, but you need to begin slowly, learning to walk before you run. If you are over fifty, badly out of shape, or suffer from diabetes, high blood pressure or heart disease, talk to your doctor first. Exercise will help you all, but do get his blessing and advice.

If you are feeling very stiff, start each exercise session with an extended warming-up period. You will find that long, slow stretching exercises will help. If you are over fifty and have not taken real exercise for some time, do stop and rest during the 20-minute session whenever you feel tired. You will find that you can do more and more each day.

Doctors in Britain are extremely concerned by the lack of exercise during old age. Most of us slow down from the age of thirty onwards, and by the fifties and sixties many people today lead sedentary lives. They should learn a lesson from Madge Sharples, the oldest female marathon runner in the country. She took up real exercise for the first time when she was already in her sixties, and five years later she claims to feel younger, more energetic and much happier.

There is a great deal of research to back her claims. It has been found that the ageing heart has a tendency to stiffen, to take longer to contract and to spend less time relaxed. But all three problems can be overcome by getting involved in a moderate exercise regime like mine. Bone mineral density also tends to decline after the menopause, but research in Finland has suggested that this fall-off can be delayed by exercise. And the body benefits in many other ways. It has been found from several studies that older people who exercise have a 'functional' age well below their actual years.

It is a consoling, cheering thought that we have so much control over our health, and that by using exercise as preventive medicine, we can delay our decline.

4 The Drinking Plan

Scientists have come to the rescue of everyone who likes to drink in moderation, whether it is a little wine with dinner every night, or regular social lubrication in the pub. It now seems that teetotallers have been proved wrong, because researchers believe that it is healthier to drink the equivalent of two glasses of wine a day than to drink no alcohol at all.

Moderate drinkers appear to live longer than both non-drinkers and heavy drinkers. Before we get too excited about this news however, I should point out that only 6% of men in England and Wales actually describe themselves as non-drinkers, and the number of people who drink heavily is increasing.

We have all heard far more about the dangers of extreme drinking than we have about the disadvantages of not drinking at all. Anyone who regularly drinks too much, runs the risk of suffering from personality changes, liver cirrhosis, impotence and brain shrinkage, which can cause loss of memory and verbal performance. There are some indications that heavy drinking increases the risk of certain cancers, and pregnant women should be aware that alcohol in excess puts the unborn baby at risk too.

The medical advantages of moderate drinking have been debated for many years. It may seem paradoxical that anyone's life could be shortened by the absence of alcohol, which we all know can be a toxic substance. But it does seem likely that abstaining from alcohol could increase your chances of heart disease.

One recent study, which found that half a bottle of wine a day could really mean 'your good health', was carried out by scientists at Bristol University. They measured the levels of HDL, a substance which helps to protect against heart disease, in normal people before and after drinking half a bottle of wine a day for six weeks.

The HDL levels rose significantly while the alcohol was being used, which provided further evidence that moderate alcohol intake could be associated with a decreased incidence of heart disease. The same study also seemed to show that half a bottle of wine might protect against gallstone formation. It is suggested by some scientists that the relaxing effect of alcohol could be another advantage, because it reduces stress and the diseases associated with it.

Other drinks which are regularly studied by scientists include coffee, tea and soft drinks, because they contain caffeine, which is the most popular and widely consumed drug in the world. It is found in 63 species of plants, including coffee beans, tea leaves and the cola nut, and it has been used because of its stimulant properties for centuries. The ancient Chinese got their lift from tea, while Ethiopians chewed coffee beans mixed with fat to prepare for battle.

Anxiety over caffeine did not surface until the Victorian times, when someone claimed that tea was 'an enfeebler of the frame, an engenderer of effeminacy and laziness, a debaucher of youth and a maker of misery for old age'.

Scientists have still not sorted out the truth about caffeine, but it is definitely a potent drug. It travels quickly through the bloodstream, reaching most parts of the body within five minutes. It increases the body's metabolic rate, as well as the output of urine and stomach acid. It is thought to make the muscles of the heart constrict, although it relaxes the muscles of the bronchial tubes.

You can become dependent on caffeine, and it can

give you sleep problems when drunk in excess. In one study, three or four cups of coffee in the evening caused several periods of sleeplessness during the night. It is thought that caffeine blocks the action of a chemical messenger called adenosine, perhaps by attaching itself to receptor sites in the brain, normally reserved for adenosine, taking it out of action.

But studies linking caffeine with human diseases are viewed with scepticism. It has been blamed for birth defects, heart disease and even cancer, but few scientists accept the findings. It is possible that caffeine can cause palpitations or abnormally fast heartbeats, and people with these symptoms would be wise to give up drinking very strong coffee, vast quantities of tea, or soft drinks in excess. One recent Norwegian study found that local people, who drank more than six cups of black coffee a day, had raised levels of cholesterol, which might increase their chances of suffering from heart disease.

But most experts conclude that concern over caffeine is exaggerated. The truth probably is that it is useful for boosting performance when you are tired, and that it is quite safe unless drunk to excess.

5 The Vitamin Plan

THE TEN VITAMIN COMMANDMENTS

1. Be careful about taking vitamins because they are sold in an uncontrolled way, and can lead to fatal overdoses.
2. Try to get most of your vitamins from your normal diet.
3. Eat fruit and vegetables which are as fresh as possible. A lettuce loses half its vitamin C within a day of being picked.
4. Cook food carefully to avoid losing the vitamins.
5. Brown rice and bread contain more vitamins than white.
6. Avoid copper cooking pots because they can destroy vitamins C and E.
7. Try not to use tinned vegetables. Frozen products are slightly better, although obviously they are not packed with vitamins like fresh foods.
8. Never soak fruit and vegetables in water. Avoid losing vitamins by washing food quickly just before cooking.
9. Never take fat-soluble vitamins that build up in the body, without following expert medical advice.
10. You will save money by buying vitamins from chemists' dispensary counters, rather than the branded versions.

More rubbish is talked about vitamins than any other of the six nutrients we need for healthy living. On the one hand, British experts tend to claim that we should be getting all the vitamins we need from a normal diet, while certain scientists in America are convinced that by taking megadoses of virtually all vitamins and minerals we can delay ageing and increase vitality.

This is the one health area where it is still extremely difficult to sort out fact from fiction. A clear scientific picture has yet to emerge. There are, however, useful points that can already be made about some vitamin supplements, and about the best way to make sure that our food is providing the range of vitamins we all need.

But, first of all, what are vitamins? They are one of six nutrients needed to maintain a stable body chemistry. The body cannot function adequately without vitamins, minerals, carbohydrates, proteins, fats and water, but because vitamins and minerals are only needed in small quantities, they are often known as micro-nutrients.

Many scientists believe that we would be much better advised to get our necessary vitamins from natural food, rather than from vitamin tablets and other supplements, because it may be that the combination of vitamins with other substances found in fruit and vegetables is important. The problem is in guaranteeing that the food we eat contains vitamins in adequate amounts.

Tests have been done on several types of food, and it has been found that vitamin levels, which are very high just after food is harvested, soon drop dramatically. Lettuce has been found to lose 50% of its vitamin C within 24 hours of being picked. Oranges which were tested, varied from having no vitamin C present when they were in the shops, to having as much as 116 mg just after being picked. The scientists who did these tests on oranges were alarmed by the results that showed some oranges with zero levels of vitamin C. It is thought that fruit which is stored for a long time, and is also injected with special preservatives, is most likely to lose vitamins.

We can do something about this by trying to make sure that we only eat fruit and vegetables that are very fresh. I grow a lot of my own vegetables, and we try to pick them only an hour or so before eating whenever this is possible. The vitamin A content has been shown to vary from 20,000 International Units in a fresh carrot, to only 70 IU in a carrot which has been stored for a long time.

Eating local food in season is not only cheaper but the vitamin content is also likely to be much higher than in expensive, imported foods. Try to buy any vegetables, fruit and salads, on the day you plan to eat them, prepare them just before the meal, and wash them quickly instead of leaving them to soak in water as many people do. Vitamins easily escape. If you do have to store fruit and vegetables, keep them in the bottom of the refrigerator. Try to avoid having to resort to frozen vegetables, but if you do, never thaw them before cooking.

Cook fruit and vegetables for the shortest possible time, in the smallest amount of water that is feasible. Steaming, and quick frying in a wok, both retain vitamins. And it is also wise to keep any water used in cooking vegetables for adding to soups. Then the vitamins are not thrown away. Eat potatoes in their skins. And as copper cooking pots can destroy vitamins C and E, use aluminium, stainless steel or enamel instead.

By following the above rules, and keeping to my Total Food Plan with its increased levels of fruit, vegetables, wholemeal products and brown rice, you should have a very satisfactory vitamin intake. But, of course, many people now do not get enough fresh foods. One study of 28,000 Americans in the 1970's showed common deficiencies of vitamins A, C and the B group. Vitamin needs vary from individual to individual, depending not only on their diet, but also on smoking, alcohol intake, exercise, age and so on. Diets high in saturated fats, for example, can increase the need for vitamin B6, because that vitamin is used to maintain fat metabolism. And alcohol is a problem when it is drunk in excess. It can prevent the absorption of vitamins that are taken in naturally with food. For that reason, some scientists recommend a double dose of vitamin B complex every day, plus a dose of multi-vitamins, for all heavy drinkers. Smoking also increases the body's needs for vitamins.

But you do have to be careful about taking vitamins. They are sold in an uncontrolled way over the counter of health food stores, chemists and some grocery chains. Many advertisements about vitamin benefits are very persuasive, and young sportsmen and women, who want to excel in their own particular events and games, are known to be especially vulnerable. They have often been told that they will only be able to push their bodies, and win events, if they take a wide range of vitamins and minerals. I have talked to teenage athletes who spend £20 a month on bizarre vitamins, and products like Royal Jelly from bees, that have never been through rigorous scientific tests. It has been known for people to die from overdoses of vitamins A, and D, which are fat soluble, and can therefore build up in the body. Fortunately vitamins C and B are water soluble, so any excess should be excreted.

Despite these problems, the Americans are vitamin crazy. They are said to spend more than two billion pounds a year on synthetic vitamins, and now they can even buy urine dipsticks, which tell them if they are excreting excess Vitamin C. The sticks change colour if the vitamin is present in the urine. Many Americans have special vitamin bathroom cabinets to put on the wall next to their general purpose bathroom cabinets, and they can buy the full range of vitamins at their local supermarkets. Overdosing is becoming a problem. Perhaps because of this, they are said to have the most expensive urine in the world.

More and more people in Britain are also taking vitamins. It is all part of the slowly-awakening interest in health. I am told that sales in health food shops were up by 15% last year. Margaret Thatcher, for example, is a well-known vitamin C fan. She believes that it keeps her fit, and increases her resistance to colds and other infections. She is always telling those around her to take vitamin C, too.

Joan Collins is a great believer in vitamins E and C, particularly E which is often called the 'Youth' or 'Sex' Vitamin. Scientists have shown that it is essential for fertility in rats, but it does not necessarily have the same effect in humans. It is, however, possible that it retards cellular ageing. Barbara Cartland has been taking vast quantities of vitamins for fifty years. Of them all, she is particularly keen on vitamin E and the mineral selenium.

SOME PUBLISHED CONCLUSIONS ON VITAMINS

VITAMIN A

It is thought to help maintain the health of our skin and the mucous membranes in our tissues. It also maintains a substance called visual purple in the eye, which is required for night vision. I do not think that it is wise to take vitamin A supplements because it is soluble in body fat, and is therefore stored in the body. Overdosing has led to fatalities. I believe that we should all be able to get enough vitamin A in natural foods. Carrots are a good source, and just one good, fresh carrot can contain 20,000 IU, which is well above our daily needs. So it is wise to eat carrots regularly, freshly grated and raw in salads, or crisply cooked in very little water.

THE VITAMIN B GROUP

Vitamin B1, or thiamine, can be found naturally in wholegrains.

Vitamin B2, Riboflavin, is found in milk and eggs.

Vitamin B3 is abundant in poultry and peanuts.

Vitamin B5, or pantothenic acid, is found in poultry, fish and wholegrains.

Vitamin B6 is in fish, walnuts and wheat germ, while B12 is found in liver.

The B group are thought to be important for our digestion, skin and nervous system, but the problem is that diets high in saturated fats can prevent the absorption of these vitamins. The Total Health Plan is, of course, low in saturated fats, and it does recommend fish and poultry, which are low in fat and high in the B vitamins. These vitamins are water soluble.

VITAMIN C

It is found in citrus fruits, tomatoes and vegetables, and is probably our most important vitamin because it is involved in so many body functions. There is some evidence that it can help to fight colds and other infections, and may help to prevent ageing and some cancers. Its benefits, however, have not been accepted by all scientists. But those who do believe in the importance of vitamin C, take more of it both during and after a cold or another type of infection. They think that the special cells in our bodies which fight disease normally have high levels of vitamin C, which drop whenever we get a virus or some other infection. They also believe that the level drops with age, as the immune system weakens. So they recommend extra vitamin C for older people, and for us all during illness. The level of vitamin C is thought to be lower in the cells of smokers, which might explain why they seem particularly susceptible to infections. It is water soluble, so any excess is excreted.

VITAMIN D

This is thought to regulate calcium and phosphate metabolism, but it is fat soluble and I do not recommend taking special supplements. It is added to milk, although the best natural source is sunlight. Vitamin D is formed on human skin by the ultra-violet light in sunlight reacting with substances found in our skin. Anyone getting normal doses of light should have enough vitamin D.

VITAMIN E

It has widespread actions in the body, and is thought to have an important role in the immune system. Two groups of mice, one given vitamin E supplements, and the other not, were exposed to the pneumonia virus. All animals without the vitamin caught pneumonia, while 60% of those on vitamin E were protected. It is found naturally in vegetable oils, wheat germ, leafy green vegetables and wholegrains. Although it is fat soluble, and can build up in the body, I do take vitamin E pills in small doses. It is, however, important to use only the newest, freshest pills. They do not keep well.

VITAMINS AND AGEING

One theory about why we age and become more susceptible to disease is called the free-radical theory. Certain scientists working in this field believe that although oxygen is vital, it has one disadvantage of producing toxic by-products called free-radicals which can damage our genetic material called DNA, our cell membranes, and our immune system. They claim that this damage ages us, and makes us more prone to infections.

But, during our evolution, it is thought that the body developed the mechanism to use various nutri-ents, like vitamins C and E and the mineral selenium, as free-radical controllers, or antioxidants. These are thought to help prevent damage to our DNA and immune system. Research has shown that mice given antioxidants were more vigorous and less diseased.

Some people have begun to take selenium in the

hope that it will protect them against free-radical damage. But it must be taken with great care, because it is toxic. It has been known for people to overdose just by breathing the fumes of copying machines, which can contain selenium.

VITAMIN DOSES

There is very little agreement about how much of each vitamin we all need. The official recommended daily vitamin allowances in Britain, for example, are far lower than the recommended allowances in America. And some scientists are saying that even the American figures are far too low, because they are only enough for preventing deficiency diseases and not for keeping people at the peak of health or for preventing them from ageing. They also say that you must increase doses if you smoke, or drink more than two glasses of wine, or the equivalent, a day.

One vitamin expert in America has published his recommended minimum doses, which exceed previous recommendations. They are:
Vitamin E — 200 IU, Selenium 25 micrograms, Vitamin A — 2000 IU, C — 1000 mg, D — 200 IU, E — 200 IU.

Some people are taking vitamins in these vast doses but few scientists would recommend it. We still do not know enough about the long-term effects of taking large amounts of vitamins. The situation is confused in Britain. On the one hand, a major report on nutrition, the 1983 Proposals for Nutritional Guidelines for Health Education in Britain, said that the body can adapt to higher intakes of vitamins, either by reducing their absorption or by increasing their excretion. The exceptions the report mentioned were vitamins A and D, which can build up in the body because they are fat soluble. But it advised ensuring minimum intake and not worrying about higher intakes.

Despite this the British recommended levels for vitamins are lower than those in countries like America and Russia. And our 30-year-old rule requiring the milling industry to put back into white flour vital nutrients removed by milling, may be ended, to save the industry about £5 million a year. This is being considered despite opposition from leading nutritionists, including DHSS advisors. Experts worry that old people and many others in Britain will have a lower intake of thiamine than the DHSS recommended level, unless thiamine in white bread is replaced.

One answer, recommended by my Total Health Plan, of course, is to eat wholemeal bread because it remains full of goodness. And eating the fresh fruit and vegetable levels advised by my plan, we should all be getting adequate supplies of vitamins. But I still give my family one multi-vitamin tablet a day as a sort of insurance policy. Each tablet contains 2000 IU vitamin A, 200 IU of D, and 25 mg of C. In the winter, or when we have infections, we take an extra 50 mg of vitamin C, and I take a small dose of vitamin E. I cannot recommend them for other people, however, because the scientific evidence is still under dispute.

There has been American research, listed in the report *Diet, Nutrition and Cancer*, which suggested that vitamins C, E and A might possibly offer protection against this disease, and a recent Japanese study suggested that vitamins E and C did both act as antioxidants, protecting our body cells against damage. After using a chemical system to check the behaviour of vitamins in the laboratory, the scientists advised that we should take 60 mg of vitamin C a day to remain healthy. Before more is known, however, we are left to make our own vitamin decisions.

6 The Anti-Stress Plan

THE TEN ANTI-STRESS COMMANDMENTS

1. Learn short-term relaxation methods, so that your body and mind can temporarily go limp.
2. Exercise regularly to produce natural opiates in the brain which make you feel high.
3. Eat well to avoid body chemistry extremes which lead to stress.
4. Discover your own perfect, personal method of unwinding when the world gets you down.
5. Make gradual changes in your lifestyle to combat stress.
6. Talk through persistent problems with someone close.
7. Perform a periodical emotional audit to identify problems.
8. Learn to control your work, so that it is kept in perspective.
9. Take a brief holiday or rest from routine if the pressures are high.
10. If stress is a regular, debilitating part of your life, learn how to alter your response to it by using my relaxation procedure.

Stress is often described dramatically as one of 'the killer-diseases of modern life'. It has been blamed for causing heart attacks, cancer and other diseases. But, unfortunately, we do not completely understand stress and its implications, although it is thought that, like good wine, a little of it can be good for us, but that taken to extremes it clouds our judgement and destroys our health.

Fortunately we can do something about it. It has been shown that regular exercise reduces stress, partly because exercise produces natural opiates in the brain, called beta-endorphins, which make us feel better and happier. Sensible eating habits also help. By following my Total Food Plan you avoid the extremes of body chemistry that can lead to stress.

Short-term relaxation also has a lot to be said for it. This has long been practised in certain guises in Eastern Societies, but for us it basically means putting our feet up for 10 minutes, or soaking in a bath. Anything, in fact, which allows us to close our eyes, think nice thoughts and allows the body and mind to go limp. It is a skill that improves with practice. Do not under-rate its importance.

When you are feeling particularly stressed, because of overwork or a personal problem, you will need to find a way of unwinding over a longer period. And one of the best forms of long-term relaxation is to get involved in some kind of activity you really enjoy. Some people find that taking a holiday which is quite remote from their normal life is the best way to reduce stress. Sport, or some type of vigorous activity, helps those who need an outlet for aggression and nervous tensions. I find that one wonderful way of achieving physical and mental release is to go on a long country walk, well away from city traffic, crowds and buildings. By doing this regularly, I find that London life no longer gets me down.

You may decide that you need to change your life-style to combat stress, but do not try to do it overnight. If you think that you can suddenly stop smoking, take exercise and eat more healthily, you are kidding yourself. You must make the changes gradually, or your resolve will fade within a week. Phase out stress-inducing habits one at a time, or you could find them ganging up on you, leaving you feeling very depressed.

If you realise that you have got persistent problems, do not keep them to yourself. If you talk them out with someone close to you, it will help you to solve them realistically, and so reduce stress. It can help to perform a periodical emotional audit, identifying both your priorities and the pressure points in your life.

Stress can be reduced if you find time to get involved in a regular activity which you really enjoy, and which is not at all related to your day-to-day life. If you work, take more control of it, so that it does not take control of you. Never create artificial deadlines, and take a brief holiday periodically when the pressures are high, just to prove to yourself that you are not indispensable. Maintain control by occasionally relinquishing it to others by delegation. Try to step back and look at your work from afar. Then you can keep it in perspective and perhaps learn to pace yourself better so that you do not suffer from overwork and neuroses about work problems that can lead to stress.

That advice may help you to be positive about stress, and it should remove some of the causes of anxiety. But it will never be possible to change every cause of stress, be it environmental like crowded roads or aircraft noise, or personal like the death of a close friend or a major emotional problem. We can, however alter our response to this stress.

The sort of people who most need to learn the art of relaxation are those self-motivated, hard-driving types who often seem impatient, restless and incapable of letting the world go by. They may have very rigid posture and use a lot of quick, darting movements. They have to try hard to suppress turbulent emotions.

It is, however, very difficult to feel deeply emotional or excited when your muscles are completely relaxed, which is why people under stress are taught to concentrate on parts of the body which suffer more acute muscular tension, like the shoulders, the neck and face muscles, the diaphragm and rib cage.

Few of us are stressed enough to need to use relaxation techniques. But, for those who do have a problem, the following advice will be useful. Try to achieve complete relaxation twice every 24 hours, once during the day to relieve tension in the muscles and refresh yourself in general, and then again immediately before going to sleep. This should help you to sleep deeply.

THE RELAXATION PROCEDURE

1. Find a comfortable position lying on the floor with cushions under both head and knees, so that your spine is resting on the ground. Let your legs roll out slightly, and have your arms at your side, palms down. Your head should be to one side, with your shoulders on the floor. Remove distractions, so take the phone off the hook.
2. Concentrate on your breathing for two minutes, so that the natural body rhythm removes any distracting thoughts.
3. Then for another two minutes, slightly lengthen the period of each exhalation. Do this gently to begin relaxing the muscles in the chest area.
4. Feel the sensation of heaviness in all parts of the body in sequence, starting with the arms, then the shoulders, spine, hips and legs.
5. For about a minute allow your stomach to 'sink' slowly through to your lower back.
6. Swallow gently and allow your jaw and whole face to 'drop' for a minute.
7. Experience a warm, floating sensation in different parts of your body.

8. Then finish with a long period of relaxation for between three and ten minutes. Concentrate on your breathing again if you feel distracted. Breathe deeply and stretch parts of your body.

So what sort of evidence is there that, by removing stress from our lives, we might be healthier and live longer? Well there is direct evidence from animal experiments that stress can cause cancer. Scientists in Seattle implanted tumours into identical mice, then subjected some to moderate stress. They were rotated in their cages for periods of time. The control mice were put in other cages with little noise, the right amount of company and no handling. Most of the stressed mice died from cancer, while more of the low-stress mice were able to combat it.

We humans are in particular danger from stress at certain times in our lives. Retirement is one time, especially for men, and the death of a partner is another. One scientist has monitored the immune system of surviving partners, and has found that for several months the stress affects our ability to fight disease. It is quite common for deaths to occur in twos for this reason.

7 Cooking For Health

Organise your meals around my Total Food Plan, and you will soon find that by eating more fresh vegetables, fruits, brown rice, wholemeal bread, and potatoes in their skins, that the amount of saturated fats and protein in your diet will be reduced dramatically.

It is easy to replace butters, lards and other animal fats with polyunsaturates. The final dish will taste almost the same. It is also possible to use low-fat cheeses in the place of more traditional types in most recipes. And low-fat natural yoghurt will often substitute for cream. Many cakes, flans, pies and pizzas can be made with wholemeal flour.

Planning meat meals often seems the most difficult. But it soon becomes a habit to buy the less fatty cuts like pork and lamb fillet, and the types of meat and poultry which are naturally fairly low in saturated fat, like game, poultry and offal. Try to eat fresh fish once a week, and either limit yourself to five meat and fish meals a week, or spread the protein content through more meals by using recipes that only need a small quantity of fish or meat. Bolognese sauce, pizzas, and many recipes from the Far East fall into this category. All my recipes are for four people.

RECIPES WHICH ARE LOW IN MEAT

My own healthy eating plan relies very heavily on one recipe. It is a tasty Bolognese sauce, intended for spaghetti, but modified to form the basis of many other dishes. It is used in lasagne, cannelloni, and when mixed with rice, extra herbs and sometimes nuts, I also rely on it for stuffing green peppers, vine leaves, cabbage and aubergine halves. With red beans, cumin and chilli added, it can make a quick chilli con carne. And, because it contains a lot of vegetables and only a little meat, it is perfect for the Total Health Plan.

BOLOGNESE SAUCE

    2 cloves garlic
    2 onions
    ½ lb mushrooms
    2 carrots
    2 14oz tins tomatoes, or the equivalent of fresh
        tomatoes when in season
    2 bay leaves
    large pinch of oregano
    black pepper to taste
    4 tablespoons tomato purée
    ½ lb very lean mince
    little left over red wine or stock
    3 tablespoons sunflower oil

Soften chopped onion in hot oil. Add crushed garlic, grated carrot and finely chopped mushrooms. Add the meat and allow it to brown gently. Add all the ingredients and simmer gently for about 1 hour.

STUFFED CABBAGE LEAVES

    2 cups Bolognese sauce
    4 cups cooked brown rice
    8 medium size sound cabbage leaves
    8 mushrooms
    1 small carton plain low-fat yoghurt
    1 teaspoon mixed herbs
    1 teaspoon paprika
    1 cup beef stock

Blanch cabbage leaves and drain. Mix sauce, rice, herbs and paprika. Divide between the leaves, push a mushroom into the middle of each and roll up, tucking in the ends. Put close together in a dish, pour over yoghurt and stock. Cover and cook in moderate oven for 1 hour. Serve with potatoes in skins and tomato salad.

CHILLI CON CARNE

    To 1 pint bowlful of Bolognese sauce, add
    2 bowls boiled red beans
    1 teaspoon powdered cumin
    4 tablespoons chilli powder (This depends on its
        strength. Some chilli powder is very hot. So
        start by adding 1 teaspoon and build up the
        strength)

Simmer for ½ hour. This is better if made the day before eating. Serve in taco shells or on tostadas, which are made with ground corn, and sold in supermarkets like Safeways under the 'Old El Paso' label. Also serve green salad and brown rice.

CHICKEN

Chicken and turkey are both low in fat, but many of the traditional recipes for them do include cream. There are, however, refreshing methods of using chicken and turkey with yoghurt, lemon, Indian spices or crisp vegetables. Chicken breast is extremely useful for vegetable-based Far Eastern recipes cooked quickly in the wok.

SPICEY CHICKEN

    4 chicken joints
    10 oz plain yoghurt
    2 teaspoons ground coriander
    2 teaspoons ground cumin
    ½ teaspoon ground cardamom
    2 cloves garlic

Mix the spices, crushed garlic and yoghurt. Cover chicken pieces and leave for as long as possible, overnight if you have planned ahead, then grill for about ½ hour and serve with brown rice.

CHINESE CHICKEN WITH GREEN PEPPERS

    4 chicken breasts cut into strips
    4 green peppers cut into small pieces
    2 teaspoons cornflour
    1 teaspoon corn or sunflower oil
    1 teaspoon soy sauce

For Quick Frying:
    3 tablespoons corn or sunflower oil
    2 cloves crushed garlic
    1 small sliced ginger root

Put chicken pieces in bowl with cornflour, toss well and then add oil and soy sauce. Prepare peppers. Heat oil in wok, cook peppers in the hot oil for 3 minutes, then add chicken pieces and fry together for 4 minutes. Serve with brown rice.

GARLIC CHICKEN

1 average sized chicken cut into 4 pieces
2 tablespoons sunflower oil
pepper
20 cloves garlic
1 lemon

Heat oil. Rub chicken with lemon, season with pepper and add to oil with the garlic. Keep turning and cook for about half an hour, by which time the chicken should be nicely browned, and the garlic golden but still tender inside. Serve with crunchy lettuce or endive.

OFFAL

This is low in fat, economical and nourishing. Here are two of my favourites.

KIDNEYS WITH LEMON GARLIC

8 lambs kidneys
1 tablespoon sunflower oil
4 large cloves garlic
juice of one lemon and black pepper

Skin and core the kidneys before cutting into ½ inch pieces. Chop garlic and fry both in hot oil, with pepper, for about 5 minutes. Add lemon juice and serve as the juices run out of the kidney. This is good on a bed of fresh spinach, or if preferred, with brown rice and salad.

CALF'S LIVER WITH ORANGE

    1 onion
    2 cloves garlic
    2 tablespoons flour
    black pepper
    dry mustard
    cayenne
    8 small slices liver
    2 tablespoons sunflower oil
    cup of stock
    a little red wine
    parsley
    thyme
    1 orange sliced

Chop onion and crush garlic. Add a pinch of mustard, cayenne and black pepper to flour. Roll liver in it. Fry in oil. Take out and keep warm. Now add onion and garlic to juices and oil. Cook slowly until golden. Add stock, wine and herbs. Boil up and spoon over liver. Serve with brown rice, garnish with orange.

OTHER MEAT

If you want to eat meat like beef, lamb and pork, do not choose very fatty cuts. If you want to grill chops, cut off the surplus fat, and remember that pork, lamb and beef fillet have less fat than many other cuts.

PORK FILLET JUNIPER-STYLE

This not only has the advantage of using a cut of pork which is comparatively free from fat, it is also quick to cook and tastes very special.

>   1 large whole pork fillet
>   10 juniper berries
>   a little margarine or oil — high in poly-unsaturates
>   pepper
>   dry sherry

Cut the pork into round slices ½ inch thick, and beat them flat. Crush the juniper berries and put a little on each piece of pork with freshly ground black pepper. Heat margarine or oil in pan, fry the pork on each side for about 2 minutes, then pour a little sherry over to mix with juices in pan. Serve with potatoes in their skin, and green vegetables or salad.

LAMB FILLET KEBABS

>   1lb fillet of lamb
>   4 tomatoes
>   1 sweet pepper cubed
>   8 pieces of onion

Meat Marinade:

>   1 cup sunflower oil
>   juice of 1 lemon
>   1 chopped onion
>   2 bay leaves
>   2 teaspoons oregano
>   pepper

Mix and marinade meat for 2 hours or more. Drain meat, put on skewers (alternately with vegetables if preferred) and grill for 8 to 10 minutes. Serve with rice and salad.

GAME

All game has a minimum of saturated fat, so eat it whenever possible. Hare and rabbit can be quite cheap in season.

MUSTARD RABBIT

>1 good rabbit cut into pieces
>2 tablespoons flour
>black pepper
>3 tablespoons sunflower oil
>1 onion
>mixed herbs
>1 glass white wine
>1 cup chicken stock
>2 teaspoons French mustard
>1 teaspoon English mustard
>small carton plain low-fat yoghurt

Roll rabbit in flour. Season and brown in oil. Add chopped onion and herbs, wine and stock, and simmer until tender. Take out rabbit, add mustards and yoghurt to pan. Simmer sauce until right consistency, add rabbit to heat through and serve.

JUGGED HARE

This is a dinner party special, which uses a marinade to make the hare less rich and less dry.

1 hare jointed
2 tablespoons sunflower oil
4 glasses wine vinegar
2 onions
2 carrots
¼ lb mushrooms
2 sticks celery
2 cloves garlic
pinch mace
1 bay leaf
pepper
1 lemon
pinch powdered cloves
2 tablespoons redcurrant jelly
Port
chopped parsley

Marinade hare in wine vinegar for 24 hours. Drain, dry and brown in oil. Put in casserole, and then fry vegetables in the oil. Add to hare with stock, mace, cloves, herbs, garlic, lemon juice and a strip of the rind. Cook casserole in moderate oven for 2 hours, then reduce temperature to low and cook for another 1-2 hours. Reduce liquid, add port and redcurrant jelly. Serve hare with sauce poured over and garnished with fresh parsley. Serve with potatoes in skins, crisp green vegetables — and some extra redcurrant jelly (home-made if possible).

FISH

Learn to love more fish. It has gone out of favour in Britain because so much of it is now frozen and tasteless. Try to support any local fishmonger who has a good range of fresh fish, crabs, scallops, mussels and prawns.

MACKEREL STUFFED WITH DATES

This healthy fish makes a special meal when cooked by this Moroccan method.

> 2 large mackerel
> ½ lb fresh or soft dried dates
> 2 oz chopped almonds
> 3 tablespoons cooked rice
> 1 teaspoon sugar
> ½ teaspoon ground cinnamon
> black pepper
> ground ginger
> 2 tablespoons margarine
> sunflower oil
> small chopped onion

Wash and clean the fish. Slit open its belly and remove any bones you can. Stone the dates and stuff them with a mixture of almonds, rice, cinnamon and a pinch of pepper and ginger — all kneaded with the margarine to keep the mixture together. Rub the fish with oil, ginger and pepper. Fill with dates. Put on foil, sprinkle with chopped onion, wrap up and seal the foil. Bake in moderate oven for 15 minutes per lb. Unwrap, allow the fish to become crisp and brown. Serve dusted with cinnamon.

MUSSELS

Mussels are cheap, tasty and fat-free. Avoid the classic French recipes which use cream. They can be excellent cooked more simply, with the juices mopped up with wholemeal bread.

MOULES MARINIERE

About 40 mussels
large onion
2 tablespoons chopped parsley
sprig of thyme
1 bay leaf
freshly ground black pepper
2 glasses white wine
a little margarine or oil

Cook onion in hot margarine or oil until transparent. Add wine and herbs and simmer for 10 minutes. After washing and scraping the mussels, add to wine in saucepan, cover with lid and steam until all the shells open. Put mussels in large bowl, reduce liquid to half and pour over. Garnish with fresh parsley and serve with bread.

BROWN RICE

Long grain natural rice and brown rice can both now be bought cheaply from most supermarkets. Use long grain if you need a white rice. It has more flavour and nutritive value than polished white rice.

Brown rice contains protein, and is rich in vitamins and minerals. It is the best choice to make for most rice dishes, but does take longer to cook than other types of rice. Wash in several waters, picking out any hard bits and floating husks. Cover with about 1 inch of cold water, bring to boil and cook for about ½ hour. It should then be soft, with all the water absorbed.

It is also good fried.

FRIED RICE

1 cup brown or long grain rice
2 tablespoons sunflower oil
1 bay leaf
1 chopped onion
pepper (add 1 teaspoon turmeric and/or 3 cloves
   to make a change in flavour)

Fry chopped onion until transparent, add rice, stirring all the time for about 5 minutes. Pour boiling water to cover the rice and add seasoning and herbs. Cook very slowly and carefully for about 30 minutes. If you are serving with Indian dishes, turmeric is excellent.

IDEAS FOR SALAD LUNCHES AND FIRST COURSES

HUMMUS

This salad is well-known outside the Middle East, where it originates. It is an excellent appetizer with wholemeal toast or pitta bread (a wholemeal version is now sold by Safeway's and Sainsbury's supermarkets). It is also useful for light salad lunches.

> 6 oz chick peas soaked overnight
> juice of 3 lemons
> 3 cloves garlic
> 1 tablespoon sunflower oil
> 1 teaspoon paprika
> 1 tablespoon chopped parsley

Boil chick peas in fresh water for about 1 hour. Drain, set aside a few whole ones for garnishing, and reduce the rest to a puree, using liquidiser, food processor or sieve, gradually adding the lemon juice and garlic. (A quarter pint of tahini paste can be added now if liked.) Pour into serving dish and dribble a little red paprika mixed with oil over the surface. Sprinkle with chopped parsley and whole chick peas.

TARAMASALATA

> 2 slices brown bread
> 8 oz smoked cod's roe
> 1 clove garlic
> ¼ pint sunflower oil
> 2 tablespoons lemon juice
> 3 tablespoons yoghurt
> pepper
> black olives and parsley for garnish

Transform bread into crumbs in a food processor or by another method. Add lemon juice and leave to soak. After about ten minutes blend this with the roe and garlic until smooth. Gradually add the oil so that the mixture emulsifies, then gradually add the yoghurt. Season with pepper and garnish with black olives and parsley. Serve with pitta bread or wholemeal toast.

This dish, hummus, vegetable flans and dishes like large tomatoes stuffed with low-fat cottage cheese make superb lunches with side salads.

SPINACH FLAN

I make this with wholemeal pastry to the following recipe:

Wholemeal Shortcrust

> 8 oz flour
> 2 teaspoons baking powder
> 2 oz margarine
> 2 oz vegetable fat
> 2 tablespoons water

Rub fats into the flour and baking powder mix until the mixture looks like fine breadcrumbs, then add water, mix and roll as usual. Bake blind in moderate oven in a flan.

This does not have the same texture as pastry made with white flour. It can be crumbly and a little difficult to handle. But well made, it tastes quite delicious. Use Allinson's, Prewett's, Sam Mayall's or any good supermarket own-brand wholemeal flour.

Spinach Filling

> 1 lb spinach
> 2 tablespoons margarine
> freshly ground black pepper
> small pinch salt
> ½ lb low-fat cottage cheese
> 1 large beaten egg
> 1 oz parmesan cheese
> 6 tablespoons plain yoghurt
> freshly grated nutmeg

Cook spinach with seasoning and margarine. Drain and then mix with cottage cheese, egg, yoghurt and nutmeg. Put in flan, sprinkle parmesan on top and bake in a moderate oven for 30 minutes.

ITALIAN FLAN

I also make a lighter version of a pizza using whole-meal pastry. Again, line a flan dish, bake blind and then fill with the following.

Pizza filling

>   1 large chopped onion
>   2 crushed cloves garlic
>   2 tablespoons sunflower oil
>   large pinch oregano to taste
>   black pepper
>   1 14 oz tin tomatoes or 1 lb fresh
>   3 tablespoons tomato puree
>   for decoration: a few black olives
>   anchovy fillets
>   sliced Italian cheese

Soften the onion and garlic in oil, add tomatoes and seasoning, cook for several minutes and then thicken with tomato puree. Pour into flan case. Decorate the top with cheese, anchovies and olives and cook in a moderate oven for about 30 minutes.

TUNA AND KIDNEY BEAN SALAD

>   large tin of tuna
>   large tin red kidney beans
>   1 onion
>   salad dressing
>   fresh herb — parsley or chervil — for garnish

Mix the tuna chunks with the drained red beans. Slice the onion into rings, spread on top, garnish with chopped fresh herbs and pour on a good salad dressing — make your own with oil and vinegar and whatever herbs you prefer

This can be made within minutes for a quick lunch snack or first course.

PUDDINGS

There are too many delicious pudding recipes to go into here but I did think it useful to include this yoghurt-based recipe as so many people make the mistake of thinking that if it is yoghurt again it must be boring.

ORANGE DELIGHT

20 oz natural yoghurt
3 large oranges
1 lemon
good tablespoon dark, aromatic honey

Grate the oranges and lemon into the yoghurt. Leave one orange to slice finely the following day and add the juice of the other oranges and lemon, plus the honey, to the yoghurt. Mix well and keep in the refrigerator overnight so that the flavours blend well together and the pudding settles into a creamy consistency. Put into bowls, arrange orange segments on top and serve.

CAKES AND BISCUITS

There are now dozens of successful recipes for making many kinds of cakes and biscuits with wholewheat flour, whole oats and so on. We do not eat traditional tea so we are not very keen on cakes in my family but I do find this recipe useful.

Oat Slices

>3 oz whole oats
>4 oz wholewheat flour
>1½ oz brown sugar
>4 oz margarine
>¾ teaspoon baking powder
>6 oz pre-soaked dried apricots

Put the dry ingredients into a bowl and rub in margarine. Put half the mixture in a greased oblong tin, press to form a base, arrange apricot filling on top, then cover with the rest of the mixture. Press down firmly and bake for 30 to 40 minutes in a moderate oven. Cool and cut into slices.

8 Shopping For Total Health

The signs that we are shopping for health are encouraging. Recent figures on food consumption, from the Ministry of Agriculture, Fisheries and Food, show that we are buying more meats which are low in saturated fats, that we are eating fewer eggs, that we are moving from butter towards margarines and cooking oils, and that fresh fruit and vegetables are becoming increasingly popular.

Health food shop sales were up by 15% last year, and other stores are showing more interest in high fibre and low fat, sugar and salt products. In late 1983 and 1984 Boots opened Food Centres in some of their shops, selling items which are healthy. Far more supermarket chains are offering better products too. The difference, of course, is that in Boots Food Centres, and Health Food Shops, customers know that everything on the shelves has been chosen because it is thought to have health advantages, while in a supermarket you have got to sort out the wholemeal bread from the sliced white, and you have got to know which vegetable oils are best to choose for health.

We have not yet gone as far as one Danish Supermarket chain, which marks healthy foods in a distinctive way. The director of its research laboratory believes shops should really push health at their customers. He wants people to buy a wider variety of foods, and he looks forward to the day when shops will have alternative brands, like low-fat liver sausage and sugarless baby foods, sitting on the shelves alongside traditional brands. He would like to see these 'alternatives' marketed more aggressively and given the best positions on the supermarket shelves. He believes that one day we could even see supermarkets divided at the entrance with 'turn left for cancer and heart disease; turn right for a healthy life.'

In Britain, supermarket customers have to find their own way by choosing stores which offer a wide range of healthy products. Surely it might even pay supermarkets to push health in the long-term, because their customers may live longer and be still shopping while rival store's customers could be lying in hospital beds. It is an interesting thought at least.

I have been checking out some of the larger stores to see what they are offering.

THE BOOTS FOOD CENTRES are a particularly interesting new development. They have excellent food fact sheets, and give a free computer diet analysis. You feed in your typical food intake, and the computer tells you how far you are going in achieving a balanced, healthy diet.

The centres encourage the idea of a diet high in carbohydrates, with Boots wholemeal flour, muesli, fresh brown bread of several kinds, and Real Growth Farmers Brown Rice. There is a whole range of products high in dietary fibre, called Second Nature brans, cereals, pastas, biscuits and flour. Jordan's muesli, Allinson's Bran Plus, Prewett's products, Kellogg's Bran Buds and All Bran, and Granose Soya bran are all sold.

In the Low-Fat section there are skimmed milks, low-fat Cheddar and Cheshire cheeses, yoghurts and crispbreads. There are vegetable fat products including Boots sunflower, soya and corn oils, various salad dressings and margarines. Vitamins and minerals are provided in health drinks, Boots Vita Food and vitamin pill ranges. And there is a very wide range of pro-

94

ducts which are low in sodium, including salt substitutes, special bread, low-salt cereals, crackers, snacks like tortillas, baked beans and many sauces.

SAFEWAY SUPERMARKETS have a good range of extremely fresh and interesting fruits, herbs and vegetables. There is a good choice of whole wheat products, including fresh pastas, and a fairly normal range of low-fat products.

WAITROSE has become known for the freshness of its foods. The majority of home grown salads and vegetables are picked and packed 24 hours before delivery, which is the same lead time as produce on sale in wholesale markets. Many of them are cooled after picking and delivered under refrigeration. At no point is the fresh fish frozen. It is selected only from inshore boats which ensures that it is delivered within 24 hours. White fish is sold within one day of delivery and smoked varieties within two days.

Waitrose sells five types of own-brand cooking oils which are low in saturated fat, including sunflower, safflower and corn oil. They stock goats milk yoghurts as well as fresh goats milk, skimmed milk and other low-fat yoghurts. They have their own-brand low-sugar jams, including apricot, blackcurrant, damson, black cherry, raspberry, strawberry and morello cherry, as well as low-sugar marmalade and special jams for diabetics.

There is plenty of choice in the high fibre breakfast cereal section from Quaker, Meadow Farm, Kellogg's and Waitrose. Several high-fibre biscuits, crispbreads and flours are stocked. Jordan's, Allinson's, McDougall's and Waitrose brands are all sold. You can buy brown rice, wholewheat spaghetti and lasagne, as well as wholemeal baps, rolls, burger buns and loaves. Waitrose stocks pulses like kidney beans, haricots and chick peas, both canned and dried, as well as fresh juices and canned fruit in natural juices. Salt substitutes will be stocked soon.

TESCO branches increasingly stock a good range of high-fibre, low-fat, and low-sugar products. They produce data sheets on the content of their foods, including cholesterol, fibre, vitamin and carbohydrate levels.

ASDA have an enormous selection of margarines and oils which are low in saturated fats. They have a good salad selection, which is helpful for anyone following my Total Health Plan, and two low-sodium salt substitutes are now being tested. You can buy low-sugar products at Asda, and a whole range of high-fibre foods, including whole wheat pasta, good flour, bread and dozens of breakfast cereals, many of which are also low in sugar.

SAINSBURY'S have their own brand of sunflower and corn oils, as well as sunflower margarine and a low-fat spread. The range of high-fibre breakfast cereals is wide, and wholemeal spaghetti, macaroni, bread, cakes and biscuits can be found. Skimmed milk soft cheese is sold along with other low-fat products like yoghurt. Fruit and vegetables are delivered within one day of being picked.

It is obvious that the large supermarket chains are selling far more 'health foods' than they did a year or so ago. Small Health Food Stores are obviously another source of Total Health Plan ingredients, although prices may be a good bit higher. These are some of the names to look out for, wherever you shop:

HIGH-FIBRE: Boots Second Nature range, including lasagne, spaghetti, flour, wheatgerm, bran biscuits, crispbread, muesli and other cereals. Jordan's products, Allinson's, Prewett's and Kellogg's Bran Buds and All Bran. Quaker Harvest Crunch and oat products, Meadow Farm Toasted Bran, Bran Plus,

Crunchy Bran, Cheshire Wholefoods products and Beemax. Foxes Oat cookies and bran biscuits, Ideal Bran crispbread, Ryking Fibre Plus crispbread, Nabisco Bran Crunchies, Energen Brancrisp, Krisprolls and Quaker and Jordan's crunch bars. Record wholewheat pasta. Boots Real Growth Farmers wheatmeal flour. Brown bread from Hovis, Windmill, Vitbe and Allinson.

LOW-SUGAR: Waitrose low-sugar jams and marmalade, diabetic jams and biscuits by Prewett, Scott, Simpson and Serionian Jams. No-sugar muesli from Sunwheel, Life and Health, and Frutifort.

LOW-FAT: Dairy produce from Eden Vale, Ski, St. Ivel, Flora and Express Dairies. Tendale low-fat Cheddar and Cheshire cheese, Express semi-skimmed milk, UHT skimmed milk, Boots and Cadbury's dried skimmed milk, Eden Vale cottage cheese. Alfonal make oils and margarine which are high in polyunsaturates.

LOW-SALT: Ruthmol and Lo Salt make salt substitutes, Gilbert's produce Biosalt, and Hugli's vegetable stock cubes are useful. Boots Food Centres also stock Rite Diet low-sodium bread, Health Valley 'Instead of Salt', stoned wheat crackers, several low-salt cereals, 'no salt' tomato sauce, vegetarian chilli, Boston baked beans, mild chilli, spicy chilli, Bellisimo, mustard with herbs, herb crackers, sesame crackers and tortilla strips.

9 Aerobic Exercises At Home

These simple exercises to do at home are aimed at everyone who has neither the time, money nor inclination for public workouts at health clubs, dance classes or swimming pools. Do them in sequence for about 20 minutes, either first thing in the morning or before eating a large meal. Many people like to do them when they wake up, before taking a shower and getting on with their day, but there are also advantages in exercising after work. Aerobics, done to music, can relieve tensions built up during the day.

Choose a spot in your home where there is plenty of space for swinging arms and legs. Use a folded blanket or large towel for lying on, and wear an old tracksuit or leotard. Choose music with a steady, easy beat. You will find that the exercises are far more fun, and even easier, than when they are done in silence.

As with all other aerobic exercises start slowly and end slowly, but in the middle, for at least 10 minutes, you need to push yourself fairly hard. Let pain be a guide as to how much to do. The old belief that 'it will not do you any good unless it hurts' is RUBBISH, and very dangerous for anyone who is unfit. You must never push yourself beyond what feels comfortable. Looseness and suppleness will come gradually, and you will soon find yourself being able to push yourself a little harder every day.

When you first start, and you are not familiar with these exercises, do them in silence. This is to avoid the danger of trying to rush through something to keep up with the music, and straining or tearing a muscle. But once you know them well, choose music you really like. And enjoy yourself.

One word of warning for the unfit people who are not at all familiar with this sort of exercise. You have to do them properly to benefit from them, and to avoid damage to joints and muscles. If you feel at all confused by any of these exercises, try going to an aerobic exercise class, just once, to try them out under expert supervision. Then, once you feel confident about them, you will be able to use them regularly at home to feel better, fitter and happier.

WARMING-UP

This is just as essential as with other forms of exercise, for exactly the same reasons. Make sure you feel warm. If not, run up and down the stairs or run on the spot.

Start standing up and do 10 SHOULDER LIFTS, which involve lifting your left shoulder up to your ear for one beat, followed by dropping the left shoulder as you raise the right one for one beat.

Then do 6 HEAD ROLLS, 3 in each direction. Swing your head to the side for one beat, then rotate it backwards so that your chin stretches to the ceiling, rotate it to the left for one beat, then drop your head forward. Do them slowly to start with — it is easy to crick your neck.

Next, 10 ARM STRETCHES, breathing in as you raise your arms sideways above your head; stretch hard, then breathe out as you drop your arms.

For the following exercise, actually touch your toes if you find it easy, otherwise just stretch down. TOUCH YOUR TOES — or STRETCH from a standing position with legs straight and together 10 times. Then, standing with your feet slightly apart, STRETCH EACH ARM down the side of your body as far as it will go. Again, do it 10 times, alternating the arms. When stretching sideways, keep the body in a straight line. It will not be effective if your head and upper body come forward as you do it.

STRETCH YOUR HAMSTRINGS by standing with your feet apart and, bending your knees, put your hands on the floor in front of you. Straighten your legs and then bend your knees to each beat, keeping your hands on the floor if you can manage it. Try to do it 10 times. If you are fit, you should find this fairly easy. Anyone who is unfit, should be careful with this one.

End the warm-up period by doing a BODY ROLL-UP. Start with your feet apart, legs straight and arms and head hanging down limply. Slowly roll up to standing erect. Now you are ready for the REAL exercise session.

AEROBIC EXERCISES should be done while breathing regularly and deeply. Start by RUNNING ON THE SPOT for 30 beats of music, then run for 10 beats, lifting your heels high behind you, then PRANCE for another 10 beats which means lifting your knees as high as possible in front of you.

Do 20 LEG SWINGS. Jump, land on one foot and swing the other leg and both arms out towards the other side. Run on the spot again for 15 beats. Then end this section by doing two more BODY ROLL-UPS.

Now, LEG EXERCISES. Lie down on your left side, and lie out in a straight line with your legs stretched and lift your right leg up then down until it is about 2 inches above your left leg. Repeat 10 times then turn over and exercise your left leg in the same way.

Still lying on your side, first on your left, bend your right knee in towards your stomach before stretching it right out again, in line with the left leg, and finally lifting the right leg straight up. Do this 20 times and repeat with the left leg.

Lying on your back, raise your right leg towards your head, keeping it straight, and pull it towards you with both hands 5 times. Repeat with the left leg.

Then stand up to do ARM EXERCISES. Hold your arms straight by your side and circle both arms forward like a windmill for 15 beats; then circle then backwards. Still standing with the knees straight, raise both your elbows out to the side as far as possible, bending the lower arm in. Then straighten your arms out to shoulder height, forming a T. Repeat to 15 beats of music.

WAIST AND STOMACH EXERCISES are badly needed by many of us. Start this section of the exercise session by standing up straight, legs slightly apart. Push down and out with your right arm, bending your left elbow up as far as it will go. Let your head fall to the right. Then stand upright and repeat the exercise 20 times; then do the same with the left, always breathing out as you push down and in as you straighten up. 10 times with each arm is enough if you are unfit.

Next, feet apart and knees lightly bent, hold your elbows and twist your body to the right for 10 beats and then to the left.

Your STOMACH MUSCLES will benefit from that old favourite exercise where you lie on your back, fold

101

your arms behind the head and your legs straight. Now lift your head and upper back off the floor by using the muscles in your abdomen — not your arms. Lift and relax back 20 times, if you are fit. Now, lie straight and lift your legs up until they are at right angles to your body. Repeat this, still with your arms folded behind your head, and lift your head and upper back off the floor 10 times. Then lie out flat again and lift your feet off the floor very slightly. Hold for 2 beats, then lower to the floor. Do this 20 times.

Now, begin to RELAX. Hug your knees to your chest for 10 beats. Then sit up straight, legs together straight in front of you and grab your toes, ankles or calves. Flex your feet until the heels lift. Pull your head and shoulders down as far as you can go. Hold for 10 beats.

COOL DOWN by lying out flat, relaxing your muscles for 10 beats, followed by hugging your knees to your chest again for 10 beats, before lying flat again.

TRADITIONAL EXERCISES

Some men, who want to exercise at home, think that aerobic movements done to music seem effeminate. So for those who want more traditional exercises, try the following for 20 minutes. But remember to breathe regularly and freely throughout all the movements to benefit the lungs and heart.

1. Run on the spot, lifting the knees high every so often.

2. Do stride jumps, raising your arms straight out to the side as your feet touch the floor, first together, then apart.

3. Stand, feet astride and arms stretched out sideways. Turn trunk to one side and bend down to touch the opposite ankle with the other arm upwards and backwards. Return to original position and repeat with the opposite arm.

4. Step up on to a bench 12 or 14″ above the ground. Lead with the left foot, following immediately by the right. Step down again with the left. This should be a continuous action and keep going for 30 seconds. After a short pause, repeat, leading with the right foot.

5. Neck rotation. Drop your head on your chest, circle over the left shoulder, backwards and upwards and down on to the right shoulder. Repeat, circling over the right shoulder.

6. Squat thrusts. Crouch with your hands on the floor, slightly forwards and outside your feet. Jump left leg backwards to its full extent and then bring it forward again to the original position, while at the same time jumping the right leg backwards. Alternate the leg movements continuously for 20 thrusts. The arms hold the bodyweight.

7. Knee hugging. Stand with feet together. Raise one leg and pull the knee close to the chest. Lower and repeat with the other leg.

8. Press ups. Start by lying full stretch on your stomach then raise yourself to a supported postion with the arms half bent. Straighten then half bend then straighten alternately.

9. Standing with the feet slightly apart, clasp hands across chest and then pull shoulders outwards and forwards as strongly as possible. Relax and repeat.

STOMACH EXERCISES

Very few of us have perfectly flat and firm stomachs. I

have therefore included some extra abdominal exercises which can be done on their own every day for those flabby muscles which need extra attention.

1. Lie on your back, neck resting comfortably, with your feet held under wall bars or a piece of furniture. Raise yourself slowly to a sitting position. Drop back and repeat several times. The number depends on fitness and health. Once you feel uncomfortable, stop.

2. Lying on your back, with arms stretched on top of your body and resting on your thighs, pull in your chin and slowly raise yourself until your fingers reach your knees. Drop back and repeat.

3. Lying on your back, neck resting comfortably, raise your legs, bend your knees slightly and then straighten your legs and slowly lower them.

4. Sit on the floor or bed with one knee raised and that foot off the ground. Place both hands on the top of the knee and push downwards to push the knee away from the body while you try and resist the movement by drawing the knee towards the chest.

5. Sit on the floor or bed with both knees raised and feet off the ground. Place hands on knees and push forward as if trying to straighten the legs.

6. Lying on your back with legs slightly raised and crossed, press upper leg down and lower leg upwards. Change position of legs and repeat.

10 One Week In My Total Health Plan

SUNDAY

My week started unhealthily with my normal Sunday morning weakness — a traditional English *breakfast*. I had half a grapefruit without sugar; grilled bacon, kidney, tomato and fried egg; one slice wholemeal bread and two cups of coffee with milk but no sugar.

I really enjoyed my breakfast, with no feeling of guilt, because for the rest of the week, my first meal of the day will be frugal.

Exercise: It's a lovely day so I decide to bicycle through the lanes of Gloucestershire for an hour. It has five gears which makes the going easier and I arrive back to face one of the greatest challenges of the week for the Total Health Plan —

Sunday lunch. We go to a party given by friends who run a restaurant. This time it is to celebrate the christening of their second daughter, Laura. Fortunately, both for my palate and the THP, there are plenty of salads and other dishes which do not break the ten commandments. I eat a delicious prawn and chicken dish, with a green pasta recipe and salads made of crisp vegetables like cauliflower. I follow this with a raspberry and nut pudding — and notice that my two sons seem to sample most of the half dozen or so desserts. Two gin and tonics and a glass of wine mean I have already exceeded my ideal alcohol limit.

In the evening, I have a simple wholemeal bread sandwich — and another glass of wine. It is the end of a
marvellous day.

MONDAY

This is a more typical day which starts as normal with
a brisk walk for my dog Sam. He is an Australian
terrier but, despite his short legs, we get round the
local park and golf course at a good pace. I then go to
the local pool for a 20 minute swim. In a good week, I
go to the pool on Mondays and Thursdays, the two
days of the week when I always wash my hair anyway.

Breakfast follows: half a grapefruit, one slice wholemeal bread with polyunsaturated margarine and
home-made marmalade with two cups of coffee with
milk.

Lunch is in the BBC canteen where the salads are a
little predictable but the taste fresh and good. I choose
hummus, fresh tomatoes and grated raw carrot with a
glass of water followed by a cup of coffee.

Dinner is particularly interesting tonight. We grow
a lot of our own vegetables and at this time of the year
— early autumn — we have a very wide choice. Our lettuce and endive are excellent so we have a first course
which uses both mixed for a Caesar salad. Our quince
tree is full of fruit this year and I tracked down a Greek
dish which added quince to pork. This is a delicate way
of cooking pork fillets with slices of quince and a few
herbs. I serve it with potatoes in their skins and
spinach.

This week I use up all the spare quince, left after
making our usual quince jelly, to produce a dozen jars
full of spiced quince. This is a new recipe for me but it
dates from the 18th century and is said to be excellent

106

with pork and poultry. Having peeled and sliced far too many quinces, I cook and store the remainder in a liquid made of wine vinegar, coriander seeds, sugar and water. Dinner ended, by the way, with sliced fresh oranges and preserved ginger — washed down with two glasses of red wine. We do not have coffee in the evening.

TUESDAY

My normal 20-minute dog walk is followed by a *breakfast* of the juice of two oranges, two slices of wholemeal toast with low-sugar jam and two cups of coffee.

Lunch is taramasalata with a green salad and coffee.

Dinner is corn on the cob followed by stuffed tomatoes (I give the recipe in this book), brown rice and salad. The children then have fruit but we just enjoy two glasses of wine — or was it three?

WEDNESDAY

Normal walk with Sam and then for *breakfast* I have green figs, toast and coffee. When I get to the office, I climb the four flights of stairs as usual instead of using the lift.

Lunch is cottage cheese, beansprout salad and coffee.

Dinner is at home with friends. We have spinach soup followed by chille con carne (recipe given) served on cornmeal tostadas with brown rice, endive, green pepper and tomato salads. We finish with plums cooked in wine and garnished with toasted almonds. Our friends drink coffee and we all drink a lot of wine.

107

THURSDAY

I walk Sam and swim before *breakfast* when I eat grapefruit, toast, a boiled egg and two cups of coffee. I am working on a live television show in the studio and at *lunch* I eat unhealthily on a pork chop, apple sauce and pumpkin. The chop is fatty and I wish I had my usual boring salad. We had a much fresher tasting *dinner* of avocado, served with chopped pepper, spring onions and parsley in dressing, followed by lamb fillet kebab (recipe included) with a courgette and tomato casserole. This excellent dish is from Elizabeth David's book, *French Provincial Cooking*. We do not have pudding and coffee, as usual, but we do have our wine.

FRIDAY

An interesting day as we are eating out at a restaurant for a special celebration. We go to Odin's and I notice the menu is full of dishes that My Total Health Plan would happily recommend. I eat chicken pâté with spiced pears as a first course, followed by lean slices of duck served in a beautiful sauce with braised shallots and radishes. This comes with a large selection of crisp, fresh vegetables. I then have an illegal chocolate pudding. Wine and coffee are drunk. As the rest of the day was frugal with grapefruit and coffee for *breakfast* and a salad sandwich made with brown bread for *lunch*, I do not worry about the sugarful pudding.

SATURDAY

This means time for a longer and more attractive walk. It is a quiet day with a salad *lunch* and fresh pasta in a home-made tomato sauce with lots of endive salad for *dinner*. We have vegetable soup as a first course and a pudding made from blackberries.

This has been a fairly typical week. But as I have not been filming, I have been able to resist those pub lunches which do stretch my Food Plan to its limits — and I have not had my traditional Sunday lunch which often contains a lot of saturated fat. So, it has been healthy as far as my food is concerned and I have taken enough exercise although I have not had time for one of my favourite five-or-more mile country walks. Perhaps next week?

I now end each week feeling far more energetic than I did a year ago, before my Total Health Plan had been born. I have done the hard work for you, by sifting through all the scientific evidence on exercise, food, alcohol and vitamins. You are left with the easy part, the part I have enjoyed and benefited from myself over the past year — THE SIMPLEST, MOST SENSIBLE HEALTH PLAN in existence. Use it to modify your lifestyle and you will find you enjoy your life more. If you follow my painless, moderate Total Health Plan — you will be able to live longer, without killing yourself.

THE POCKET HOLIDAY DOCTOR
by Caroline Chapman and Caroline Lucas BM BcH

All the do's and don'ts for a healthy holiday . . .

How to keep the family free from holiday hazards . . .

How to cope with sickness, diarrhoea, sunburn, bites, fever, etc . . .

Zero hour – when to recognise that you *must* have a doctor, and how to find one in any language . . .

One of the authors of THE POCKET HOLIDAY DOCTOR, Caroline found herself in a mother's nightmare. In an idyllic holiday home, her ten-year-old child developed a temperature of 103° and had diarrhoea so severe that she was passing blood. They had no transport. The nearest telephone was half a mile away, the nearest doctor ten miles and he couldn't speak English.

There and then Caroline Chapman vowed that if her daughter pulled through, she would write a book offering practical advice.

Here, from Caroline Chapman and Dr Caroline Lucas, is a book for emergencies of all kinds, from the sting of a jelly fish, to a possible outbreak of cholera.

0 552 12195 9 £1.25

SEXUAL HEALTH AND FITNESS FOR WOMEN
by Kathryn Lance and Maria Agardy

A NEW WAY TO SEXUAL AND REPRODUCTIVE
WELL-BEING

This book tells you how to:

* Be more responsive sexually
* Have more and better orgasms
* Relieve menstrual pain and pre-menstrual tension
* Achieve easier childbirth and recovery

and at the same time, how to:

* Flatten your stomach
* Streamline your bottom
* Firm your inner thighs
* Build muscles that fight backache

and much more. This is the first book, written by women
for women, to tell you everything you need to know about
strengthening your pelvic girdle. General exercise won't
do it. But this proven three-phase programme WILL!

0 552 99011 6   £1.95

A SELECTION OF HEALTH, PHYSICAL FITNESS AND FAMILY LIFE BOOKS AVAILABLE FROM CORGI

While every effort is made to keep prices low, it is sometimes necessary to increase prices at short notice. Corgi Books reserve the right to show new retail prices on covers which may differ from those previously advertised in the text or elsewhere.

The prices shown below were correct at the time of going to press.

☐ 20279 0	**DR ATKINS' NUTRITION BREAKTHROUGH**	*Robert Atkins M.D.*	£1.50
☐ 22776 9	**THE ALEXANDER TECHNIQUE**	*Sarah Barker*	£1.75
☐ 01435 8	**JANE BODY'S NUTRITION BOOK**	*Jane Brody*	£4.95
☐ 99033 7	**ARTHRITIS**	*Rachel Carr*	£1.95
☐ 10336 5	**THE MAGIC OF HONEY**	*Barbara Cartland*	£1.50
☐ 12195 9	**THE POCKET HOLIDAY DOCTOR**	*Caroline Chapman & Dr. Caroline Lucas*	£1.25
☐ 20669 9	**HEART RISK BOOK**	*Aram V. Chobanian, Lorraine Liviglio, Patrick Reilly*	£1.25
☐ 01293 2	**ANATOMY OF AN ILLNESS**	*Norman Cousins*	£1.95
☐ 20641 9	**WOMAN'S BODY: AN OWNER'S MANUAL (Illus.)**	*The Diagram Group*	£1.95
☐ 10515 5	**MAN'S BODY: AN OWNER'S MANUAL (Illus.)**	*The Diagram Group*	£1.35
☐ 23147 2	**WHICH VITAMINS DO YOU NEED?**	*Martin Ebon*	£1.75
☐ 99044 2	**THE HERPES BOOK**	*Richard Hamilton M.D.*	£2.95
☐ 13812 X	**RICHARD HITTLEMAN'S YOGA FOR TOTAL FITNESS**	*Richard Hittleman*	£1.50
☐ 23475 7	**RICHARD HITTLEMAN'S GUIDE TO YOGA MEDITATION**	*Richard Hittleman*	£1.75
☐ 23544 3	**RICHARD HITTLEMAN'S INTRODUCTION TO YOGA (Illus.)**	*Richard Hittleman*	£1.75
☐ 22869 2	**WEIGHT CONTROL THROUGH YOGA (Illus.)**	*Richard Hittleman*	£1.25
☐ 12158 4	**THE BEVERLY HILLS EXERCISE BOOK**	*Roberta Krech*	£1.75
☐ 99011 6	**SEXUAL HEALTH AND FITNESS FOR WOMEN**	*Kathryn Lance & Maria Agardy*	£1.95
☐ 01409 9	**INFANT MASSAGE**	*Vimala Schneider*	£1.95

ORDER FORM

All these books are available at your book shop or newsagent, or can be ordered direct from the publisher. Just tick the titles you want and fill in the form below.

CORGI BOOKS, Cash Sales Department, P.O. Box 11, Falmouth, Cornwall.

Please send cheque or postal order, no currency.

Please allow cost of book(s) plus the following for postage and packing:

U.K. Customers—Allow 45p for the first book, 20p for the second book and 14p for each additional book ordered, to a maximum charge of £1.63.

B.F.P.O. and Eire—Allow 45p for the first book, 20p for the second book plus 14p per copy for the next seven books, thereafter 8p per book.

Overseas Customers—Allow 75p for the first book and 21p per copy for each additional book.

NAME (Block Letters) ....

ADDRESS ....

....